*From My*

# *My*
# Job Interview
### *with*
# God

*Pamela K. Thomas*

*My*

# Job Interview

*with*

# God

*Nursing: The Perfect Job*

## Pamela K. Thomas

Mill City Press

Mill City Press
555 Winderley Pl, Suite 225
Maitland, FL 32751
407.339.4217
www.millcitypress.net

Unless otherwise indicated, Scripture quotations taken from the (VERSIONS USED)

Paperback ISBN-13: 978-1-66288-940-0
Ebook ISBN-13: 978-1-66288-941-7

# *BOOK DEDICATION TO*

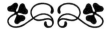

My FATHER, who was the living definition of unconditional love (I miss you);

My MOTHER, from whom I inherited a strong desire to learn and how to be strong and self-sufficient;

My CHILDREN, Jennifer and David, who are among my most precious gifts and biggest cheerleaders;

My HUSBAND, Steve, who has read a library of books and seen more streamed movies than I can count in order for me to pursue my love of nursing. He never once complained when what I made best for dinner was reservations.

Thank you to my wonderful family who have been completely supportive of my dreams, accepted late birthday cards, all-night study sessions, and my occasional roller-coaster emotions (those words are my evaluation).

Writing is now my new career and exciting adventure. Each of you have helped make my dreams come true. For all of this and so much more, thank you.

I LOVE YOU ALL

# CONTENTS

❧❧❧❧

# *INTRODUCTION*

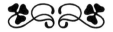

**LIFE IS THE** most precious gift we are ever given. But this amazing gift is just the beginning of our story of life.

Upon the birth of a newborn, family traits are promptly claimed and celebrated by the parents. How deliberately they instantly point out the noticeable visible look-alike qualities. This exercise is a validation of pride and connection. A type of ownership. Reality sets in with the visible likeness that proves this baby is not "just a baby," but a "mini me" of sorts, and it is thrilling. While children continue to maintain or develop more defined family traits, they quickly begin to become somewhat unique by developing their individual personality as well. Similar to a flower, they are unique and fragile and strong and vulnerable and pliable and influenced by their environment. Each life is influenced by experiences, both planned and unplanned, thus, becoming their personal road map of life. Everyone will experience life in their diverse ways as they travel through the twists and turns as they know and live it. This journey is labeled "living life."

Daily, our paths and personalities are molded and influenced by our surroundings. Our curiosity inspires growth, opening the windows of opportunities in life. Each and every individual will have many opportunities to choose their direction while following their own heart and desires, becoming a unique self-portrait of who and what we are. However, truth is, there will be unforeseen, as well as unwelcome, events that will modify the ability to choose a perfect pathway. Learning to overcome these tests and diversions in life are the building blocks of learning problem solving. We devote time to asking ourselves how to conquer obstacles, not lamenting why it happened. We strive to move beyond in order to achieve our desired outcomes.

Stages of life are what is referred to as the process of development, growth, and aging. In finding our way, the one thing that is guaranteed is it will not always be without difficulty or extra effort. Detours are on every road of life, and we can gain valuable knowledge along the way to learn to make better decisions. Importantly, we acquire knowledge on how to navigate around obstacles. Tough days are just as important as good ones. Not as much fun, but we can count them as a success if we learn from our mistakes. These trials can give us the biggest smiles and satisfaction as we learn to manage life in a positive manner. This is considered getting smarter with our choices.

Happiness and success are what we strive to ultimately achieve. But along the way, in order to know joy, it is necessary to experience sadness. Life needs balance for us to understand and appreciate it to its fullest. It is good to let sadness in. This helps shine a bright light on the wealth of joy. To know success is to have experienced failure. Before long, we gain a trust within ourselves and believe that, if need be, our courses can be altered and steered in a preferred and positive direction. When we experience moments that result in loss of faith in ourselves we judge life as not fair. Then, we put our positive thinking cap on and see it also offers options on how we can achieve more favorable results. Seek and you will be rewarded. Be amenable to change. Be observant to opportunities and quiet your minds so you can take in all that surrounds you. Just running forward with your head down at full speed, you will most assuredly run into a brick wall, not the optimal outcome you had planned.

Let's give credit where credit is due. A sense of humor affords us the ability to laugh at ourselves, which is never a bad thing. Okay, face it, we all make mistakes, so why not own them, learn and move on? Look for the laugh lines on people's faces and make them your friends. They are the real ones and also the ones that will accept you and understand you for who you truly are, flaws and all. Look for that amazing person that is willing to make tomorrow better than today. What a gift we can give ourselves. I say, challenge accepted.

Being perfect, I've heard, is boring. Strive to avoid boredom. Others will feel more comfortable around people whom have been through failure and survived. A person who is flawed will have scars from life's challenges; this person has managed to pull through not by standing with their back to the challenge but by facing their challenge head on. Scars show you've fought the battles and therefore understand the hardships others have endured. I've been there, done that, survived that. To be loved requires being vulnerable and real. These scars are the reminders of life's battles we have won. Not all scars are visible but are evident once you become engaged with others. They become apparent when compassion is exhibited. These are the real people. To be idolized is not real love. It's a photoshop picture that covers all the flaws. Thus, we are unable to feel the real, raw love that we so heartily crave and that spawns growth and purpose.

Comedians tell jokes, and people laugh. Hopefully. Well, the reason we laugh is we can relate to some of the imperfect characters, either within ourselves or others. These situations make us laugh, not just at the joke but at ourselves. This is healthy and we don't have to hide behind the ownership of these jokes. There is a wonderful acceptance for ourselves by owning them. Your friends will soon try to one-up you by telling a story about their silly faux pas. Don't make life so serious you forget to laugh and enjoy. Look at yourself every now and then in a mirror, and make a funny face. I'll bet it will make your day.

A human is one that is not immune to mistakes but can admit to needing help while learning through the process. A fulfilled life is blessed by embracing honesty. Your life journey is earned and not promised after birth. It serves as one's biggest and most rewarding efforts ever put into anything. Celebrate not only you but those whom you surround yourself with. Be an advocate and a safe house where others will feel the welcoming calm. Also know, there are a lot of underlying issues we will never figure out. We then must choose to move on and put our efforts toward other endeavors. Assuredly, each life is a personal patchwork quilt requiring stitches every day. Even the toughest speed bumps along your way, although unpleasant, offer us a jolt toward personal growth and clarity. While they are preparing us with an ability to withstand the assured battles ahead, ultimately, leading us to our intended and envisioned destination. The picture of our future is likened to finger painting, just smudges at first, but when we add more colors we can see the high lights and low lights, thus becomes a masterpiece known as "our life journey." Adjustments open opportunities that only knowledge and experience can produce.

I truly hope you enjoy your own journey and amazing adventures each and every day. Live as if you are the "special occasion" and every day is your special holiday. Make memories that will be so special you will cry many happy tears for years to come. You have a right to be proud of yourself.

# *GETTING TO KNOW THE AUTHOR*

**WHEN A PRODUCTION** company releases a movie, they begin by visually painting a vivid picture exposing the theme of the movie, commonly known as a preview. Consistently, they typically begin by revealing a teasing glimpse into the importance of the main character, setting the scene, so to speak. You become drawn into the movie and are left begging for more. We are subsequently able to instantly feel intrigued by the story and/or a character. At this point, we become engaged, while it becomes personal and the character becomes more accessible. We are then hooked.

Here is a little glimpse into the character in my book. That character is me, portrayed along a part of the amazing journey I've been blessed to have traveled.

# *PAMELA KAY, aka*
# *JACQUELINE GAYLE*

**MY BIRTHPLACE WAS** Tampa, Florida. I grew up as Pamela Kaye. However, it was not until I was 21 and applied for a marriage license that I learned this was not my name on the birth certificate. These changes were my mother's wishes.

Birth certificate: My birth name was Jacqueline Gayle.
Name change: At two and a half years old, Pamela Kay.
Growing up: I was told my name was Pamela Kaye.

From what I was told, my mother wanted to change my name but didn't know to what, so each week, as I found out later, she called me a different name and settled on Pamela Kay, making that the final choice. Still not satisfied, when I started school she spelled my middle name "Kaye." I found this a bit irregular while laughing many times about it. I've yet to come up with a good explanation though. Better than "Hey You", right?

My life, like yours, is and always has been full of people who have and continue to influence me. Being a kid comes with the luxury of time, the only constant being that of unexpected twists and turns. On a positive note, we can observe adults and strive to become the opposite of what we don't like. Plus, we can follow the examples of what we admire in others. Daily, we are forced to make choices. With the blessings of choice, we become active in being the personal designer of ourselves. This is our life, so we must choose wisely. Indeed, some situations are more challenging than others. Difficult moments give us an opportunity for positive personal growth. Hopefully, we will take advantage of our experiences and learn to better our life while helping others see that, through adversities, anyone can flourish. Here are some real-life examples of the important contributing characters in my abbreviated story of life through my eyes.

# *MY FATHER*

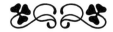

**THERE IS A** reason I started with him first. He was kind, gentle, and caring. He took his roles of husband and father to heart. At an early age I grasped how comforting it was to have a father like him. Consistently, he was a loyal and hard worker without complaint. Honestly, I can only recall a few occasions when his serious voice would flare up. During those rare moments, I saw not an angry man but a determined man who was standing up for his convictions and faith. Consistently, he was considerate, understanding, and loving. But there was a clear-cut line that was never to be crossed, and he never wavered.

He was not afraid to voice his opinion and would step up to back it up with why he felt that way. I respected those boundaries and admired the strength he exhibited in staying true to his passion and feelings. His rules were founded in decency and honesty. Plus, in true character, he never expected more from people than he demanded of himself. That was the man I knew and the person that made me very proud to be his daughter. He was that regular 7 a.m.–4:00 p.m. guy, early to work, punctual, rarely called off sick, honest, and trustworthy.

My dad had a really fun side too. He loved plaids and colorful sports jackets. He was always the life of the party. The funniest thing was him letting Mom color his silver hair with green dye for St. Pat's Day. He loved to square dance. He also played the piano and organ without a lesson in his life. A natural rhythm that filled his soul. He could out-whistle any bird. I considered this a talent and often requested a performance. It didn't take much to entertain me, but he always made me laugh and proud to be his daughter.

As his child, I felt loved and protected. My appreciation and practice of respect was also acquired from his tough love. This combination gave me a clear understanding of the steadfast rules of the house and of life. As any child, I unwittingly, or at times knowingly, did test the line. Plus, I'm positive I did come up short of his expectations upon a few occasions.

Discipline was usually enforced with a stern conversation reaffirming behavior rules. This was the serious side of our conversation. Once he felt I understood the meaning of our talks, he flashed his encouraging smile and a wink that made it all better. I could then return to life with knowing exactly what I had done wrong and promptly put that on my Do Not Do Again List. Other forms of discipline were reserved for serious offenses. I rarely experienced the advanced forms of discipline from my father but knew these were available if he needed to use them, which he would if the gravity of the offense demanded it.

Disappointing my father truly was the worst punishment of all. I felt as if I was showing him I didn't love him enough to behave. His softness after the lecture I took seriously would dispel any doubt I felt of being loved. What a gift.

I learned the meaning of respect at a very early age through his honesty, direction, and love. I always knew what I had done wrong. Lying deserved an even stronger punishment and humiliation. This was the way I learned responsibility. Doing wrong wasn't just about being wrong but about recognizing it and admitting wrong and correcting the behavior. Nothing wrong

4

with being wrong, just take responsibility and learn. Greatest lesson to this day.

My father passed away on Father's Day. I've always felt this was special and a validation to honor him as an amazing Father.

# MY MOTHER

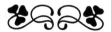

**SHE WAS STRONG,** controlling, domineering, and not one to lavish praise but quick to express disappointment and point out failures and flaws of others. Her judgments were not always relevant and rarely understood by the victims of her disdain. At least in the mind of a child, myself, this is what I observed and felt. Let's just say there was never a kiss and reconciliation after being reprimanded. Every child, even adult, wants to know what they did and why it's bad. But questioning her with a "What did I do wrong" would instantly result in further detention and punishment. Never question was the lesson received when talking with my mother. This was her stage, and she intended to keep it a solo performance.

I learned to think of other things while she was directing complaints and imposing sentencing.

The numerous sessions of her berating in such a condescending manner while yelling were very difficult to endure and frequently erratic, catching us off guard and confused. In contrast, I always understood why I was being punished by my father. I was deserving of every penalty he imposed. On the contrary, I rarely understood what I had done that was so heinous according to my mother. I was a fairly quiet and well-behaved child and easily self-entertained. I truly wanted to understand, but these sessions only drove me further away from her.

Mom frequently would reminded me, whether intentionally hurtful or not, how smart my siblings were. She called me the dumb child. That's the honest truth. You can take a breath now. It was okay then, and it is okay now. Something in my brain allowed me to internally laugh at her absurd statement. I had developed a mechanism to reject any ill-delivered words from her and compartmentalize them into a space that was the same as a trash can and never thought of the can again. The garbage man picked up the trash regularly. What I did know was she was absolutely correct. I'll explain. Her presentation and choice of words where sad for her to use toward a child, but I let her own them, not me.

Strangely, I became quite adept in tuning out the noise and anger in her tone. I became deaf and numb to her wild tantrums. I don't really remember being hurt by those words. In fact, I joke about it to this day. Actually, I found it to be sad for her. Furthermore, my siblings never made me feel that I was less than them in any way. I think they were more upset than I was.

Accepting my lower academic skills was not difficult in that it was a fact. Maybe I wasn't dumb, but clearly, I was not at the genius level my brother and sister were. My siblings aced every test, got every academic award, and their papers were always perfect. I was proud of both of them but also accepted and understood I was not the family scholar. Nor did I try to be something I wasn't. I had no desire to compete with them in any way. I was utterly proud of both my siblings and celebrated their victories without jealousy. I just knew my life was mine to figure out and become the best version of me that I could. Through all of this, I was a very happy child.

What became my chosen path was finding my own place to thrive. Tuning out the clamor of negativity became my specialty. Her "word noise" was like the busiest street in Manhattan at rush hour, and I mentally retreated into my mental and physical safe, quiet place. I found I could and wanted to thrive in a calm and giving environment. I knew exactly who I wanted to be as a person and was not going to let anyone capsize my hopes and dreams. My joy was found in being a cheerleader for others and finding the bright shining light outside my mother's numerous reminders of my failures, which was not a competition I could or wanted to win.

I chose to vanish from this dark room and approach my journey and desires through joyful explorations.

I wanted to enjoy life and do that which would fulfill the tranquil life I sought. I chose to have a positive attitude, grateful heart, and always tried to bring joy to the room. I needed a generous dose of laughter. My laughter bank was overdrawn and required many deposits. My business plan while still living at home was composed of thinking happy thoughts while being berated and not taking ownership of false accusations. The words, or as I called them, my "get out of jail free card plea," I'm sorry," became like a Tourette response. No meaning to them. Just obligatory before being allowed to return to real life. However, in real life—not when I was dealing with my mother's unending criticism—I was sincere and meant I'm sorry when I said these words.

After completing my chores and when I was finally old enough, I was allowed to go outside alone and play. In fact, I was basically on my own with the only rule, be home for dinner. Best day of my life when I heard my mom say that. My dreams of adventure began. I completed my chores in record time and perfectly so that no evidence of neglect could be grounds for detention. Dishes washed and put away neatly, bed made, towels hung, clothes from laundry folded, yada yada. I think this was the beginning of my OCD path. Sorry to all the others that have had to endure my tidy habits.

Being outside and free energized me. There was no yelling or drama. What I heard were birds singing and kids playing and laughing. I walked by people smiling and saying hello. I was so happy and embraced every moment. Truly, it was like being out of jail. Breathing in the fresh air of freedom was like smelling fresh bread baking, and the sound of people and life was like music from a merry-go-round. I was sure I could probably fly if I wanted. I would lie on the grass and look at the clouds. I was able to see figures that looked like children, angles, sheep, and people holding hands, to mention a few. To this day I still look at the clouds and find figures.

Without a doubt, I knew that was the day I initiated myself into a new life, a life that was going to define who I was and who I wanted to be. There was a world ready to be explored, and I was just the one to do it. All I had to do was look, and I was certain that when I saw my future, I'd know the path to pursue. My life was no longer under a microscope of that unattainable excellence measuring stick. I was free to look around and figure it out. No longer was I party to those moments when I felt smothered. I never met a stranger, I was never afraid to venture beyond the fence of life, and I never sat back to be just an observer. On the contrary, I was an adventurer at heart, looking for all the good things that made life exciting. My eyes were wide open allowing me to see numerous possibilities, and I wanted to experience all of them.

Trouble was never anything that appealed to me. I think my father was a good example, and I admired that. Plus, I continued to want him to be proud of me. To me it was like polar opposites being around anyone who engaged in bad behavior. I was too young to know what I would discover or like, but I knew it was out there for me, and I was enjoying the adventure of searching. My efforts were put into motion while having a childlike vision and being totally confident I'd discover my place. I set out like an explorer in an unknown land to find and create my destiny.

As I look back, it amazes me how confident and curious I was. I really didn't know what confidence was, but I had it. This probably comes from being naive. A common phrase I used in my life was "I can do it myself." And I did, many times. I am still not sure whether that was confidence or stubbornness. Or maybe a little of both. Figuring out how to do things on my own was so much fun. To this day, I laugh every time I say, "I can do it myself." I didn't have Google back then, but I surely would have worn it out with all my questions.

Adults were comfortable for me to be around, and many welcomed me onto their porches and into their homes. Occasionally, a cookie or piece of cake was offered, and I never refused. I'd walk up and down our sidewalk and speak to everyone along the way. Soon they would wave and say hello. I was in a world that recognized me and knew my name while treating me as someone worthy of taking time with. Day after day went by without being yelled at. To this day, I don't like yelling or sarcasm. It makes me cringe like playing a wrong note in a symphony.

Ironically my mother did me a huge favor. I did not want to conform to the mold she wanted for me. No longer was I a "third wheel" participating in her restricted designs for my life, and I was overjoyed. I had a strong desire for personal growth in almost everything except academics. My schools B's and C's were acceptable to me. Excessive energy and a strong sense of curiosity gave me a self-proclaimed authority to push the boundaries into the unknown. My stories of the life I planned for myself were safely tucked into my heart, and only I had the key to open them up and shape my future. Challenge accepted.

# SARAH AND WHISKERS

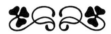

**ONE NEIGHBOR NEXT** door was referred to as the witch by several people in the neighborhood. I thought that was cruel. This theory and uneducated label was formed because of what people observed from the outside of her home. Cedar planks all weathered away from years of neglected repairs. Her home was dingy. The crevices of the siding were filled with mold and mildew. Excessively tall unmanaged trees overshadowed many shorter trees causing them to be mostly barren from leaves except at the very top. They were begging for just a little ray of sunlight, thin and tall with spindly starved twigs of branches protruding out of the lower portion on the trees. It was difficult to see the house from any angle due to the thicket of overgrown vegetation. The trees served as ladders for numerous overzealous vines. Vines also draped the house, making a dense camouflage appearance of mystery; the vines thrived over the porches and into ever crevice along with everything they could attach themselves to. Ferns loved the shade and happily grew up the tree trunks while peeking out of the vines. Boards were falling off the siding while the roof took on a calico patchwork appearance. The gutter squeezed as they dangled from their corners while flooding over onto the walkway providing the moss the moisture it needed to thrive. Dark and dreary described her home.

I spent many hours thinking about who could live in this abandoned looking home. None of my theories proved to be correct. There was no fear on my part as I was intrigued to see who lived there. Then my wish came true. I saw movement in the yard, so I proceeded to the fence to see what or who it was. I squinted through a sliver of space between a few of the vine-smothered bushes. I was embarrassed to be caught staring, but she saw me watching her.

Breaking the silence and awkward situation, I asked her what she was doing. With that, she smiled at me, probably thinking how funny it was that this little curious-about-life child started a conversation. "I'm dying yarn with these berries," she said. "Oh, that sounds fun," I told her. "I've never done that." Although I was completely unaware, this was a little rude and like inviting myself over to see how she does it. My unrelenting questions came in rapid-fire succession. She appeared only delighted to respond in a way that excited me even more. As the conversation continued, with her hand she tucked one vine over another and pushed it to the side. This gave me and her a clear view of each other.

She was as engaged in explaining her hobbies as I was in listening. I enthusiastically drank in every detail and moment she afforded me. We stood there for a good hour, talking about what the yarn was going to be used for and her loom for weaving . Her hobbies didn't end there. She went on to tell me of her love for copper hammering. Every story left me craving more. I still remember how gentle her voice was with a face to match the kindness of her heart. I was so thrilled and I suspect too forward. Never once did she show she wanted to end the conversation. She gave me her unabashed attention. She seemed delighted in my interest and had a spark of joy in being able to share her love of life. She took an interest in me while devoting her time and kindness. Her calm interaction made me feel as though my questions were grounded and valued. I was taken by her inviting and nurturing demeanor.

Then an unwelcome event occurred: my mom called me in for dinner, just as I was making a friend. Selfishly, I wanted more time to talk but nonetheless remained grateful. "Thank you, Miss . . . what is your name?" She said, "Sarah, and what is yours?" I told her Pam. "Thank you, Miss Pam, I hope we can talk again, and maybe you can come see my loom. I call my loom 'Whiskers.' Of course he had to have a name. He will look forward to playing with you." I waved bye and told her how much fun I had. She agreed, saying, "Me too." No longer was I upset I had to go in for dinner, because tomorrow I'd see her loom Whiskers. In hindsight, very presumptuous of me.

I could hardly sleep that night thinking about the Whiskers and the copper and the yarn. To me, naming her loom actually seemed normal. With curiosity, which by now should be my middle name, I peeked out the window before I tucked myself in bed. Her light was on late that night, and I imagined she was dying her yarn and hanging it to dry. Surely, she had to have it dry before we could continue our play date the next day. Another presumption.

To my dismay, Sarah was not in the yard the next day. At least not during the time I spend peering through the thick vines. Being a persistent and needy child, I went out the following day and played until I saw her peeking through the brush and waving. I rushed over to the bushes as if it were Christmas Day and asked if she had dyed her yarn. "Yes, Miss Pam, I did. It is drying over my kitchen sink." But she said she saved some for me to dye as well. "Would you like to come over and do some crafts today?" she asked. I was ready to walk right over, but she encouraged me to go in and ask my mother. I told her, "No. She is busy working." Mom worked from home. So over I went, straight through the thick of the overgrown vegetation, no thought was given to going up the walkway to her front door.

Stepping inside her home was like going through a time warp machine. Even as a child, I noted the advanced age of everything. I remember thinking how cool it was to have such huge pieces of furniture. She had two tall clocks, both in the living room facing each other on opposite walls. Within moments, I heard the cuckoo of one of them. Shortly after, the other one mimicked the same. Sarah said, "They talk to each other every hour." She purposely set on 5 minutes ahead of the other so they could talk. They too had names, Gus and Danny.

After thinking for a moment, laughter came to me so effort-lessly. Sarah said, "Silly us." Sarah was downright easy and fun to be around. It was completely possible for me to let down my guard and just be a fun-loving child. This is who I wanted to be and how I wanted to live my life. I realized that there was a place for me to fit in and enjoy the multitude of possibilities life has to offer.

All her toys and projects were piled everywhere, and the loom was even bigger than I could imagine. It looked three times as big as our church organ. First thing we need to do is learn how to dye yarn. Although that was exciting, I was anxious to play with Whiskers. That's exactly what we did after we dyed some yarn. Threading the loom with spools of yarn was complicated, but she made it fun. I got to choose four colors to weave into a place mat. She had a shelf stacked along a wall filled with any color you could imagine and more. The next step was how to pass the shuttle of thread and manipulate the organ-like pedals; she laughed at my comparison. Each pedal had a number like 1, 2, 3, 4, and they represented the color they would allow to be used. The pedal made the yarn go up and down, creating a pattern on my placemat. To be able to push down the pedals, I had to slide up to the very edge of the seat. My toes had to be in a pointed position in order for them to press down on the pedal, making it shift the yarn and create the pattern.

Patience described her in every way while gently correcting my direction with reasoning and positive reinforcement. I was thrilled with my accomplishment. I made a place mat. My very first one. I suddenly felt smart in a way that I wanted to be. This was the best day of my life, so far.

At the end of the day, I was extremely proud of the little place mat and the ability to understand the functioning of the loom's pieces and parts. When I returned home I rushed up to my room and put it in a drawer. I never showed it to my mother. I didn't want to ruin my day with being scolded for anything. Nor did I want to be prohibited from visiting her again.

This was not the only time I spent with Sarah. We talked through the vines occasionally, which always ended with, "See Ya Latter". I think it was a tie who was looking for the other one of us more often. It always seemed like seeing a long-lost friend for the first time in forever. Never once did I think it strange to be a friend of an elderly lady.

A couple of months later she invited me over to hammer a copper dish. Again, I was proud of my achievement. The fact that the dish wobbled when placed on the table didn't discount her accolades for my talent. She made me feel smart and that I did a perfect job on everything I tried. It was always difficult to leave and go home, but I didn't want my tardiness to cause me to lose my visitations with her. I made it a habit to talk to the cuckoo clock as I left. I told them thank you for talking to me and making me laugh. Sarah would hug me when I came in and when I left her house. This is the first time I knew what unselfish love felt like, other than the love from my father, and I wanted to continue to feel this way. My father gave me this kind of love, but Sarah gave me approval as a friend, and that made it unique.

As I lay in bed that night and was thinking about Sarah, my mind focused on the name-calling, "Witch," which was a common theme whenever someone referred to her. I remember how angry I was and couldn't wait to defend her the next time someone called her that.

School soon started up again after our summer break, so my time was limited. Frequently, I would see her next to the fence, as if waiting for me to come home from school. She would wave to me and ask me how school was, almost every night. It was such a sweet welcome home. I made it a habit of going to the vines each day and was overjoyed she was there most of the times. Now, I believe I was her joy too.

# BOB'S MARIONETTES

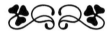

**LUCK FOR ME** didn't stop there. About a week after meeting Sarah, I ventured over to see if she was there, but she was not outside. I was disappointed but happy knowing I'd see her again soon. It was a Saturday, and the weather was really sunny, making me glad to be outside. The swing set would have to be my friend that day. Dreaming and thinking always gave me comfort. Now I can relive the fun and not have to pretend. But I still did dream a *lot*, such as what would it be like to be a bird and fly around the sky all day. My imagination and strong desires for adventure provided me with not a what-if but a when. I always felt as if anything was possible.

As I walked around the house, I saw a man in the garage next to our house. He had a light on over his workbench in the garage, and I heard the sound of drilling followed by the humming of a saw. He was making something that required wood sticks. He too had lots of machines and was practicing what appeared to be a hobby. I just stood there staring at him through the window and wondering what kind of hobby he was enjoying. There I went, curious again. It's a good thing I've learned a few more manners since then.

When he looked up and saw me staring, I waved at him and smiled. He waved back with a smile as well. Just a small eight-year-old with blonde curly hair and silly like most kids that age, waving at all the neighbors.

We had a small swing set in the backyard, where I would go to play and dream. My dreams were always there waiting for me, so I was never alone. Surprised, I heard him call to me. "Hey kiddo, what's your name?" Quickly hopping up from the swing, my legs were in forward motion rushing over to make another new friend. Wow, I thought making friends was really easy. I didn't know that making a friend meant they had to be my age. I found experienced people a lot more interesting. He was an elderly gentleman, about 60 or so, although I'm not totally sure about his age, since age is interpreted differently at the young age of eight.

"Hi, my name is Pam." "Well, I'm Bob," he stated in an uplifting tone. He had a puppet like I'd never seen before. There was a handle made of wood and strings. The puppet's mouth would open when he moved one of the big wooden popsicle-like stick. Multiple strings ran through multiple sticks, each one attached to one of the puppet's legs or arms or mouth. "Nice puppet," was my starting phrase. With a giggle, he said, "Not a puppet, dear." This made me a little confused. "I make marionettes as a hobby." He asked what my hobbies were, to which I replied, "I don't know yet, but I'm going to get one." Sounded as if I were going to put that on my grocery list to pick up next time I was in town.

"Would you like to see my workshop where I create these?" I'm sure I started walking toward the shop before I could even finish the three-letter word, yes. The workshop was fully organized, everything in its place. I remember thinking how different this was to Sarah's home. Her home was full of boxes here and there, yarn hanging from every doorway, bottles, jars, clumps of wildflowers hanging upside down from the beam across the kitchen, and baskets piled full of assorted useful play things that were precious to her. The clutter difference didn't change my feeling of being welcome in either home. We spent the day making, sanding, threading these amazing puppets, oops, marionettes. After that, I must have said that word 20 times. It made me feel quite grown-up and educated. Smart too. The thing he had in common with Sarah was his gentleness and ease, allowing me to try, and showing me how what string controlled what body part of the marionette.

My new friends gave me a certain confidence and feeling of belonging and enjoyment I never felt before from others. Bob told me I was a natural. Such a delightful comment to give to a kid. These comments and supportive moments from my two new friends totally changed my life. They gave me a sense of belief and proof in my ability to fulfill my comment, "I can do it myself." I had to ask my father what it means when someone says you are a natural, in order to confirm it was a good thing. Another fabulous day in a world I now knew had a lot to offer me, and I was ready to experience it all.

Bob continued bringing over his newest marionette creation to show me. In his other hand was always one for me to play with. At first, he gave me a simple one to operate. We had marionette conversations back and forth, pretending to be putting on a show. He started showing how to operate them one stick at a time, beginners level. Then I was a super star. According to myself. But Bob agreed, of course. I was promoted to an advanced level while using multiple lines and sticks. I learned to move knees, elbows, head, and of course mouth. We pretended they were us while we talked through them. Not sure which one of us had the most fun.

The best was yet to come, but I had no idea it could get any better. He made one with blonde hair and big puffy lips of pink and blue eyes as big as saucers. Yep, you guessed it. He named it Pam. He was hilarious. It was better than winning the blue ribbon at the fair. Not that I would know but guessed this was better. This was a phrase I had heard before, and since I was all smart and grown-up now, I wanted to use a phrase that would impress my new friends.

Several months went by and I missed Bob who had not been in his workshop. I found out that he had cancer. Our time was cut too short. That fall the unthinkable happened. I was told he passed away. This was the first time I'd faced this sort of grief. I spent the next couple of days in my bedroom, crying and being angry. None of this made any sense, and I was truly devastated.

On the way to the funeral home, I remember protesting vehemently about having to go. But my mother demanded I straighten up and behave. There was no way I could face seeing my friend in a casket. I'd never been to a funeral before, let alone one for a best friend. *Petrified* is the word that comes to mind now, but then I was just completely numb, short of breath, lost, angry, confused, abandoned, and suffering from a most unbearable loss.

Dressed, as mom told me, in my Sunday best and new black shiny shoes, I looked the part, but my face told a different story. Outside, the rain was coming down in buckets—a day that matched the dark sadness of the clouds and gave them a reason to cry. Dad parked the car and proceeded to open the car door for me, all the while tears mimicked the rain, flooding down my face in a torrential flow. This was the first time I'd ever felt betrayed by my father. Later, I understood he did not betray me. I was only trying to blame someone for my pain. How could he not see my overwhelming misery and despair?

Well, here it came, my obstinate side. My biggest defiant stunt *ever*. Even to date, I cannot think of any worse behavior than this one. The rain was coming down in sheets while my father held an umbrella over my head. He wanted to protect the curls Mom had fashioned for me that morning and my almost new pink ruffled dress. I looked up and saw the church to my left and a big nasty mud puddle to my right. Yes, you guessed it, and you are two steps ahead of me, I'm sure. Without hesitation, I dashed directly over to that big puddle behind our car, which appeared invitingly, and plopped smack down in the middle of it. My hair was soaked from the pouring rain and my dress was dripping with muddy water making me look like a little urchin. There was no possible resolve to this awkward situation.

Permanent damage had surely been done. I made my only possible choice of action since my tears were unsuccessful in convincing my parents to yield to my wish of not going into the church. I was now unfit for church. A mud puddle became my triumph. I won. Sort of. Knowing my certain fate, I was willing to take what would most assuredly be the maximum punishment that I was about to receive from both of my parents. It was worse than I thought it would be.

For the next week or so, I was unconsolably sad. Seclusion was my only friend. Overly dramatic, but it was frightening as much as it was sad. I was engulfed in the emotions of my life's first tragedy. Finally, the memories of this amazing friend began to seep into my thoughts and put a half smile on my face. No longer was I dwelling on my loss, but I started enjoying and reliving all the fun I had with him. The precious memories of our friendship were as fresh as they were the first time.

Shortly thereafter, we suddenly moved, which usually meant financial difficulties. Nevertheless, I was fortunate to take with me the memories of these special times with my neighbor friends. My only regret was not getting to say goodbye and tell them each how amazing they were and how important they were in my life.

I knew there was a world waiting for me, and it was my task to live it the best I possibly could by making good choices. My neighbors and the generous attention they showed me was the life I wanted to live. It was exhilarating to learn new things, surrounding each day and filling each moment with the love they taught me. It felt amazing to be encouraged, helped, and loved. Sarah and Bob were my springboards to become what matters to me in life: someone who cares for others. It leaves an impression that lasts a lifetime. It has left a lasting impression in my life for sure.

Giving love and joy back to others in life has given me an even greater happiness. Memories of how I felt when I was showered with love from my neighbors sparked my desire to pass on forward their same gift of kindness. Life is squandered when it is shadowed by doubt and criticism. It was my choice to reject that type environment and be the positive kid I was inside all along. My life was going to be my own canvas to paint. There are no acceptable excuses. My motto became "I can do it myself," and I set out to achieve the life that made me whole. I had a confidence that constantly nudged me to figure it out. Don't be a victim, be a student of life, celebrate your experiences, and follow your dreams. Allow and help others follow and believe in their dreams. Each one of us is unique. Like a garden, we possess a variety of different shapes and colors and fragrances, hence making life beautiful.

# THE SEARS CATALOG

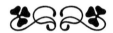

**MY ADVENTURES CONTINUED** as I was now 10 years old. It was after school when I opened the mailbox to collect our mail. Catalogs were a perfect way to dream and provided me with endless entertainment. Today there was a newly published copy of a Current Catalog. Immediately, I took it directly to my room and started my mental ordering. The pages were soon worn from turning them back and forth, circling my wants of what I wanted to order. Dreams have no budget. It never was a downer to know I'd never buy the things I had so carefully chosen. It was more like playing house and pretending to have the resources to spend if I wanted. Having things was not the thrill; it was being able to order anything I wanted. Pretending made this possible. A new catalog offering page after page of seasonal and special cards, stationery, notepads, wrapping paper, etc. I turned the pages and drooled over the pictures and read the verses on each and every card. Twice. This was the first catalog of its kind. Clever, I thought, was this concept of selling by mail.

My favorite was the Annual Sears Catalog, which always showed up right before the start of the school year. With great anticipation, I would check the mailbox daily beginning the first of July. School dress shopping meant we got to choose a few new dresses, so we anxiously awaited the appearance of their new magazine of dreams. Quickly, this event became almost as exciting as Christmas. I would go through each page so many times they all became ragged. I'd flag pages and pretend on ordering all the pretty dresses. My mom was clever with this activity, however. My sister and I were each given a budget of $25 to spend on back-to-school clothes. The budget amount was enough to purchase about four or five dresses. The prices on the dresses ranged from $3.99 to $10.99 each. If I bought one of the more expensive ones, it would be a big portion of my total allowance. I really had to want it to sacrifice almost half the money. I always opted for the less expensive dresses. Then when school came, I never really missed the $10.99 dress. This was my first hand at understanding the value of budgeting. This also was an exercise that has carried me through my life. I learned that everything was not just about the price, but it was about the value it meant to me. Did I want one dress enough to pay for the highest price dress of $10.99? Therefore, I could only get one dress instead of two dresses or perhaps three if I went with the lower priced dresses. My choice was ultimately made by choosing more dresses than being limited to fewer if I bought the $10.99 dress. It was always the cutest dress that was the highest, but I thought I'd get tired of wearing it a couple of times a week.

With the arrival of the next Sears Catalog, I was keenly aware of cost vs. my lesson on how one dress would have to replace two or three. To this day I appreciate this life lesson, while giving special kudos to my mother. There was no spending without money. Since dreaming has no budget, I continued to circle and flag while pretending to be able to buy anything I wanted. Then, I would decide on my personal value of what I wanted to spend my money on. Thoughtfully, during my second round through the catalog I crossed out all things I could truly live without.

When the Current Catalog came, I was no different. I studied each page. I circled the number of the item on each page I thought would be nice to have or at least I liked. Then, the best opportunity was stuffed halfway through the catalog: a form to fill out. This I found out was called an order form. Bold letters, appeared like a shiny object, "You Too Can Sell." This was the solution to my buying challenges. Now I had the opportunity to turn dreaming into a cash flow. What caught my eye was the catch phrase "You Too Can Sell." Thus meaning, I could order at wholesale prices and sell at retail to my customers. Cha-ching! All I had to do was submit an order form to the company and deliver the product to the customer.

My mind raced with thoughts that I was 10 without an income source. Who frets about stuff like that at 10? Yep, me. Just to have a little money in my pocket would be comforting. This is absolutely the opportunity I was waiting for. Immediately I started to practice my nonexistent sales skills, first by deciding how I would present this plea to my mother. She would be my first hurdle to achieving my financial independence. Much thought was put into my spiel. It must carry enough optimistic evidence to be persuasive. When it looked as though my well-thought-out sales pitch to my mom wasn't working, I resorted to a lame 10-year-old kid's method. I ultimately resorted to begging my mom to let me do it. As I saw she was caving a little but not yet to the yes answer I wanted, I added more promises. I think she could see I'd offered everything I could, and believe me, it took a lot of spontaneous promises and coaxing. But, I finally heard her say yes.

After successfully making my case, I darted up to my room and began putting together my sales package. Obviously, my briefcase was quite comical and juvenile. Or maybe sad would better describe it. Then came the issue of business cards. My fancy cards were handmade squares of paper handwritten with name and address, clearly having the appearance of being made by a 10-year-old. My packet was complete with the printing copies of order sheets. I signed up with the company. Saturday morning

I quickly journeyed out making my door-to-door sales pitches to the neighborhood. I had a very immature way of writing up orders, so I reasoned it made more sense to give them the forms to fill out.

As I reflect back on my "first job," I can't help but smile. Never once did I think I couldn't do this. No doubts ever crossed my mind. I was never taught that I could do anything. Maybe I just felt a sense of freedom to think and become the real me. What I know I had and still have today is an insatiable curiosity and desire to go out into the world. My customers who submitted their orders must have thought it was cute having a little kid sell stuff. Real stuff other than rocks painted in funny colors. I never thought it odd. Plus, there were some really nice things in the catalog. What also made an easy sale was a new and fresh idea to the market. My first day out I had five orders. They paid up front without hesitation. Upon completion of the sale, I reached into my sales kit, made from an expandable file folder, and pulled out one of the little squares of paper containing my name and phone number. Now all that seems impossible, but it worked. I took the money to the post office and got a money order, filled out my order sheet, and mailed it in. I was now a business kid. It was my first official entrepreneur endeavor.

Each order worked perfectly, and I delivered them with a handwritten thank-you note to each happy customer. I loved interacting with adults. I'm not sure if they wanted me to stay and chat or if I just enjoyed it so much. My questions were all about what they did and where they came from. I hung on every word and found it fascinating. The sessions usually ended with cookies, cake, milk, or pie with milk. I do remember how excited they were when I would take my dish to the sink. Once again, kudos to my mother. She was good at instilling in us values and manners. Tough lessons but most were good.

About three months later I received a new catalog with new seasonal items. Of course, out I went to canvas the neighborhood for another round of orders. I increased my customers with eight new buyers. Most of them gave me cookies and milk or hot chocolate. With each new catalog I set my feet to the pavement and sold my wares. Then after four times there was enough money to buy my Christmas presents for my family while having some extra cash for what I called my pocket money. A jelly jar became my bank, which was secured by hiding it in the back of my closet.

I was hooked and never wanted to be broke again, knowing at such an early age that it was up to me to make it happen. I truly was infected with the capitalistic bug. I may not have felt a scholastic achievement but felt a certain sense of success. There was never any praise or congratulations given to me by my mother for my tiny success as a salesperson, but my customers gave me enough praise for a lifetime. Therefore, I was well rewarded and encouraged.

# *MY FIRST REAL JOB*

**AT 14 YEARS** of age, I needed money for a cheerleading sweater and letter. I think it was $22. My mother told me we could not afford it. The possibility of not being a cheerleader was not a failure I wanted to face. I had faced this kind of bump in the road before and chose to refuse failure. To be chosen in seventh grade to be a cheerleader was a huge moment for me. People in school were nice to me, but I was never considered popular. But, to me, this felt like a welcome hug and gave me a feeling of being accepted by my classmates.

My gut instinct was to say to myself, "Don't accept no for an answer," and it was also my motivational challenge to figure it out. Again, "I can do this myself." So I pedaled my bike to a grocery store six miles away and went in to apply for a job. The manager was smiling the whole time. I thought he was pleased with me and wanted to offer me a job. As I look back, the truth was probably not the first time I was perceived as being a little young for the job application. I'm sure being a top-selling card sales gal would give me all the heads-up on how to close this sale. When he asked me why I wanted this job, I told him. At the time I didn't realize it, but again in hindsight I'm sure this was the deal closer. It was closed with nothing but honest truth. I needed a cheerleading sweater and letter and couldn't afford it, so here I am and need a job. This was not quite the way I phrased it, but putting the pieces together was easily done. I provided him with the info, and he was able to understand my plea.

After a 30-minute interview, he told me I was underage and needed the signature of a parent on the application form. I had to get the job and knew this was the way to make the sweater and letter a reality. I could work cash register on the weekends or nights after school. I would get union wages but didn't have to join and pay dues because of my age. That was $1.95/hr. Baby-sitting was 75 cents/hr. if they had multiple children. Being quick to calculate, due to my extensive sales experience, this was over two and a half times as much per hour, with a guaranteed number of hours. I figured out in one week I could pay for my sweater and letter. I got on my bike and rode home and immediately had my mom sign the consent form. Before the ink had time to dry, I was back on my bike to deliver the signed consent. I worked 20 hours a week for the next three years. Without fail I rode my bike to work and never missed a shift. I didn't get a driver's license until I was 18 years old, mainly due to having no car. Well, that and the need to stockpile some money to get other things. But I was working on changing all of that.

Upon graduation from high school I secured a full-time job at the local bank. I knew the bank manager, and he was willing to give me a chance. What a great job. As a teller I now had a steady income. My first order of business was a budget. I put a large chunk in savings every payday. I again rode my bike to work, which was only about three miles from my house. My boy-friend was in college. We had plans of getting married the next year. Halfway through the first year at the bank I bought a used Rambler American car and got a driver's license. Yes, I finally got my license. I had saved very close to the amount to totally pay for the car. Subsequently, I acquired a loan from my bank for the remainder. My plan was adhered to with perfection, and I paid the loan off throughout the following year. Now I was debt free. I was finally a big girl and making big-girl decisions.

# MARRIAGE AND DIVORCE

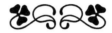

**A YEAR LATER,** I married my boyfriend of five years, who had graduated from four years of college. My focus turned to working while he attended law school. We did fairly well and remained content with our meager earnings. I do remember once collecting cans and bottles we turned in for cash, which we used to go to the local Dairy Queen. The humor was worth it. We would laugh but never felt ashamed. Obviously, money was tight, but I never felt I did without. My dreams gave me a drive to be able to look ahead and work to get there. We were on a plan for our future, and we were able to accomplish our life goals. After he graduated, we were blessed with two children, a girl and then a boy. I continued to need to work and was never able to be a stay-at-home mom. I never missed an activity or event. I was totally my children's biggest cheerleader. Being a mother was the best thing in my life and continues to be. After they each completed college they both chose their journeys and have also been blessed with a beautiful family. Pride continues to swell in my heart as I think of what amazing adults they have become.

Those speed bumps in life never quit coming, but we learned how to overcome most of them. Life has a way of altering the perfect course of our dreams. Little did I know the hardest decisions were still ahead.

Divorce was never a goal I set or expected for myself. Who would aspire to fail? My family, life, joy, and goals were sewn into the fabric of my being. I had set out to help those I loved achieve their dreams, ambitions, and always placed my focus on their achievements and well-being. For this I have no regrets. Every moment of every day, I devoted myself to them with all the love in my heart. To this day my kids remain the most important people in my life.

But now, here I was , 39 years old, divorced, sitting alone the first night in my dimly lit rental apartment. It was a second-floor walk-up to which I moved every box myself. I was literally alone. This was now called home.

The sun had almost set, and I was sitting there almost in total darkness. My choice was to wallow awhile in pity. I deserved this time of sadness and also knew I deserved better. A moment of self-approval was needed to block out the pain of what was ultimately failure. My life had become smothered with others controlling my every move. Like a rewind to my childhood. This was my burden, and there was no blame on others, as I had accepted this for years. I felt as though I had lost me. Lost was the girl that was always positive and found a way to make things happen.

It was as though there were automatic blinds over the windows that were lowering themselves, leaving me starving for a glimmer of light. The blinking clock light on the oven was the only hint of light inside the living room/kitchen. A streetlight shadow soon began to cast a small ray of light from the back bedroom window, and a streak of light was trailing down the hall into the living room, the darkness perfectly mimicking my mood. Here I sat in complete exhaustion resulting from working at warp speed like a mother robin preparing a nest for future hatchlings. Except I was just trying to survive. I was lonely, confused, afraid, sad, and empowering every possible emotion to converge upon me all at once. Motionless, I sat and took ownership of a situation that was devoid of any turnaround option. A major pity party meltdown.

After a waterfall of tears and a few outbursts of anger, I began thinking to myself and trying to apply some reasoning to my life and the sentence it had imposed upon me. There was no one else there to talk to. Or so I thought. There I was in Orlando, didn't know a single person, and was truly alone but found some comfort in hearing people in the stairway. I was crushed though by their laughter and envious of them having another person to be with.

My muse, who at times was unrelenting, as at this moment, began forcing me to listen. "Where is that person I know that can make things happen? You know the one who confidently says, 'I can do it myself, no matter what.'? Girl, you need an attitude adjustment and a job," continued my inner commonsense tough and rather intrusive and annoying muse. "Back off," I thought. "It's not been twenty-four hours yet, so cut me some slack." In order to get away from listening to all that tough love, I decided I needed to get out for a few moments. The cure for a bad attitude was a long walk and fresh air. The way I felt, I was sure I may not be home till morning.

The apartment felt cold and lonely. It didn't feel like home yet. Being distracted by other things was what I wanted and needed. Told myself not to come home until you change your attitude. I had no destination in mind, so I was being led by where the sidewalk was taking me. My thought to myself was, "Fine, who cares attitude." Just the attitude I was trying to shake. I had no plans, no map, no vision. There I was just walking off the last bit of energy my body could muster. The exact moment I thought of turning around to go back, there was a light on the corner shining down on a gas station and mini-mart. I remember thinking how bright and obnoxious that light was. It could have served as an interrogation strobe. While continuing the focus on myself, I justified that I was deserving of something I would not normally eat, but I instantly realized this was revenge eating. "Take that bad attitude!" My strike back against pain and the only control I could claim. Surely, they would have hot dogs, potato chips, beef jerky, or my choice would be a highly caloric rich candy bar. My favorite bar was an Almond Joy with a coconut center and almonds drenched in chocolate. Not the regular size but the supersize meant to share with friends. Not feeling benevolent, my plans were to totally not share or save the other half for later. There was not a shred of guilt during my overwhelming need for an Almond Joy. I felt a strong urge to challenge myself to eat it in two bites. I rationally thought of this indulgence as a serious lifesaving measure or at least it would surely change my resentful attitude toward life itself. How's that for an attitude adjustment solution. This was well-thought-out, right?

With only one step into the store, there it was, *My Future*, a newspaper. A mental flash that spontaneously registered, the Sunday newspaper was full of job ads. After my sole purchase of the paper, I abruptly returned to my apartment within half the time it took to walk to the store. Instantly, I was excited with the prospect of finding a job for my future. Distraction was placed right in front of me on a flimsy wire rack a half a step inside the little mart. My plans of soothing my anger with that candy bar were wiped from my memory. I did not even notice the counter where every imaginable candy selection was fully stocked and noticeable to even a half-blind person. But I was blinded by something else: the key to my new life. Here came that pushy girl I've known before. I can do this myself. "She's back," I said to my now focused normal self. The self-deprecation did not totally stop right then but let enough positive light through to start making a new life.

It was not until an hour later did I realize I had *no candy*, just a paper. My moving survival kit consisted of only 6 packs of microwave popcorn. But it had to do as it was my only option in staving off starvation. Yes, this is a little melodramatic. I had two bags of popcorn and consumed both of them in record speed. Now, with an enormous thirst, in my non existent survival kit was tap water. The tap water had a nasty metallic taste to it, and of course there wasn't any ice yet. The saving grace, the popcorn was butter flavored. Note to self: need groceries.

Page after page, nothing called my name. I had no formal education, even though all those I loved did. Negativity was peaking around every corner. Rejecting it with every ounce of stern fierce determination, I found the courage, allowing me to create the right opportunity to return to spoil myself with another popcorn and back to the job hunt. Being alone allowed me to lick the butter from my fingers and laugh at myself again. It had been a whole day, and this was a real breakthrough.

I thoughtfully prayed without anger or self-pity. Speaking with an open heart and in a gentle tone, I said out loud, "God, what am I going to do? And I need your help!" He knew all along and had already given me the answer. I just didn't see it yet. Just like the candy bar, I lost focus on the problem at hand and was giving into my doldrums. His answer was always right in front of me. My focus was absent, but his never was. My hungry pity party had taken my energy, which was leaning toward empty, and became an all-consuming distraction.

All the job opportunities were framed in big, fat, tall letters surrounded with attention-grabbing frames of stethoscopes, needles, and nurses hats. Don't you think he could give me a bigger clue? Such as, "HEY PAM, LOOK HERE" circled with a red sharpie! There was an extremely high demand for nurses. Each hospital was attempting to outcompete with the others. They were offering RN employment with enticing bonus options. One hospital was even offering a car with a two-year employment contract, plus a salary that would sustain my expenses. God was using every flash card to point me in the right direction. How many times can God show me the way? Once I heard, once I focused, I got it. Just like a parent who tells their kids something numerous times before it sinks in. And I thought I had a busy job raising my kids. At least they grew up and became adults. Then, God gets them back and has to deal with the complications we add to their lives, and then we expect him to solve it at the snap of a finger.

# COMMUNITY COLLEGE

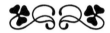

**PASSION AND DETERMINATION** were now being set into motion. Not like that girl that sat in the mud puddle but the girl that was going to walk right up and in through the door of the community college and claim my future. Now the channeled motivation fired me up while my new direction gave me an internal feeling of peace. I finally allowed my zest for life and newfound journey to bring me back to that girl that says, "I can do it." Total exhaustion could no longer be ignored since now my next life journey was set in motion. After a long shower I slipped into fresh, clean sheets with an alarm clock on the night stand set for early. As I prayed before closing my eyes to go to sleep, I felt safe and at home. God knew I appreciated his love and direction. I promised not to let him down. This was a promise I couldn't fail to keep. Then instantly, like a baby who sleeps through the night, I fell fast asleep. Confidence was once again embraced with a plan I prepared to set into motion come morning.

Confidence did not subside upon waking earlier than my alarm. It was now Monday morning, the day I will set a new life journey in motion. I dressed in a college student look, trying to downplay my age. All I lacked was a sweatshirt with the college name on the front, but I was ready to study, with an I-can-do-this attitude.

My energy level was soaring with excitement the next morning. Toast and coffee were my energy breakfast bar. Then, I promptly went to Valencia College, where I was directed to the counselor's office. There wasn't any wait for an appointment. Not one single detour flag showed up on my way. This venture showed no delays, no effort but was surprisingly easy. I knocked on the door of the counselor's office, and the counselor casually called out, "Come in." The moment I walked in, I knew this was the right decision. "Please have a seat. How can I help you?" stated the counselor. I explained that I wanted to enroll in classes to become an RN, so how and where do I begin? I turned my dreams over into his hands and never looked back.

My counselor quickly became a close and brother-like friend with whom I learned to effortlessly and countlessly rely on. He was honest with me and put me at ease. Obviously I took the title Counselor literally. I was able to throw all my frustrations of school, life, and junk at him, and he would listen to my long-winded rants. Then, when I took a breath, he would ask, "Are you done now?" I always left laughing and forgetting the purpose of my counseling session. He confided in me as well and was always encouraging me at every turn and much like my father. I never wanted to let him down. My most pressing mission, next to school, was to make him proud of me. The comforting thing was he would tell me when I was wrong. We would then talk it out and end with a mutual, warm smile.

I had no family around to confide in, so he became my mentor, who would celebrate or offer words of advice. For some odd reason his approval was only secondary to my personal pride and success. I think I convinced him I was better than I actually was. This helped me too in that it pushed me to do better than okay. I had just a few friends in the beginning and little time to develop our friendship. Plus going to school with students right out of high school wasn't the crowd I fit into or wanted to hang out with. My limited social life was enough to keep me happy. Church, Cancer Society, School Leadership Council, and an occasional social event was all I needed. These were always secondary to school. Almost every waking hour I studied, ate TV dinners, and—to my amazement—I never once questioned my ability to do this. "God, you really are my Savior." I never looked back while studying every day into the night and beyond. Once I completed my core courses, I was accepted to nursing school, where I made lots of friends and was fulfilled in many ways. The third child made it after all. My new mantra was not the original "I can do this" but rather, "I can do this myself, with God's help."

I graduated from Florida College of Health Sciences with an RN degree. The teachers and the entire support staff were absolutely the best. I definitely picked the perfect school for me. I was honored to give our student graduation speech. My class had become like a family. It was a rather small group of students, and we all supported each other. We survived study groups, listened to each other with various family issues, health problems, and remained available for one another. I did have the most amazing college friends even with the age difference between some of us. I completed school with exemplary grades and awards and was now a nurse, respected by my peers and the faculty, and being proud of my hard work was only the beginning of what was to come.

My search initially was just for a job. Never was it my future passion or dream job. But it became my dream job. God knew all along where I belonged, and he never once let me stumble. Sitting in the dark with no distractions was the most effective way for me to stop and hear past the silence. I learned to be quiet so I could feel and hear God.

People celebrate how great the nurses are and how much they have done for them, and nurses are heroes. While I am grateful for the support and recognition of being a nurse, I have a very different perspective of my career. I say, "Thank you" to my patients whom have given me a career with the most magnificent memories. "Thank you" each and every one of you for bringing me into to your lives and welcoming me as if I were family. To be able to share in your grief and joys has brought a tremendous understanding of the meaning of life. My life has been enriched and made whole because of each one of you.

I've worked in nine different hospitals, three surgical centers, and worked in three states. I worked with a nursing agency for about half of my career before becoming an employee of a local hospital. Loved every moment of it. Thank you all for the opportunity of a lifetime.

I am honored to share a small sampling of my special stories with you. Patients were never just a room number. Never a John or Jane Doe, although I have had some of those as well, but I personally gave them a name so I could relate to them. I had to know who they were to fix what they needed. We are told to look at the root cause, and to me that isn't just the disease process but rather, the whole person. The fun part is that they were all different. And so, the puzzles of nursing began. Patients are very prone to hide their pain in places that don't show. We are taught to find not just the open wounds that are evident but the pain less visible. I invite you into a few stories of my incredible journey and career as a nurse. My hope is that you will clearly see why my patients were special to me.

# *WILLOW WEDNESDAY*

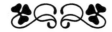

**TODAY WAS A** very exciting day for me. New job, day one. Not only was I feeling positive, but the sun was shining down and felt like a warm hug. I closed my eyes and looked up at the sky, when a brief cool breeze danced across my face. Very timely, and of course, what was the thought in my mind was, "Today is going to be a breeze." It was my nature to make the best associations possible in every situation. Wow, today is the day I begin a new adventure. I had *no* doubt it was going to be epic. Feeling quite confident and probably overly so, there I was in my neatly pressed white lab coat and scrubs, which showcased a sharp crease down the front of my pant scrubs. Later, I discovered this was a bit odd. I had what I considered a very professional appearance. Eventually, I would find out that nursing never ends the day with freshly pressed anything. Undoubtedly, I was prepared to greet every event that day with a positive attitude. My self-confidence hoisted me up as I was very assured that my knowledge would serve me well. In contrast, this first day showed me I had a lot to learn. Nope, I didn't know it all after all, as I was about to find out. Books are wonderful ground works for nurses but prove to be just baby steps. These are just a foundation and we are responsible for building the skyscraper. My self-ordained mission was, however, genuine in wanting to make a difference in the lives of others.

Another affirmation of an amazing day was the ambience in the lobby. It was brimming with laughter and giggles. A greeting far surpassing that of a red-carpet event with the spotlight focused on one person. Everyone was chanting her name, Willow. Clapping and shouting came from every corner of the large two-story-high welcoming entrance. It certainly earned its name that day. People rushed to her while hugs of greeting were freely given. Clearly, she was deserving of Hollywood celebrity status. How could one person create such a celebration? Smiles were worn from ear to ear by all who knew her. It was as if she were a long-lost friend that had made a surprise visit. The explosion of affection did not seem to subside as I walked past and glanced back to see this celebrity, Willow. She was obviously struck by the kindness of the staff. Her glance toward them was bashful and coy but showing a genuine appreciation for the attention, which permeated throughout her body. Surly she felt as though she had won the homecoming queen title. It was notable she slowed her pace as she passed by the front desk, as if to absorb every moment of her glory, obviously, well deserved. It was the most beautiful moment one could ever imagine. Oh, to be loved like that. This was nothing rehearsed, it was genuine. It was admiration from life's very foundation.

As I watched Willow's runway stride, it struck me what was really important in making a difference in the lives of others. It is a beauty from within that makes a person glow like an angel. It is a raw essence that cannot be faked. It is owned.

Willow was not tall, thin, loaded with makeup, or her hair exceptionally well styled. Rather, she sported navy blue scrubs that appeared to look like hand-me-downs. Noticeably, they were a tad too short and in all likelihood were retrieved out of the laundry basket just before leaving home. Her beauty was not altered by makeup. Makeup would be a typical practice the girls her age would be prone to wear. But, it was quickly obvious, she wore the most precious article of all, her *smile*. Her smile could light up any room on the gloomiest of days, as it did that day.

Later, I was enlightened that Willow was part of a special-needs group that came to the hospital every Wednesday to volunteer. It gave her and the rest of her group a meaningful purpose and pride. What more could anyone want? Her disability was no longer a prevailing handicap. Willow was accepted as one of the workers of the hospital, doing a job, having a purpose, and all along being loved, appreciated, and bringing special joy to others. She was given a job, and she returned an even greater gift to so many. We seldom look at reality through the eyes of others. But this day, we experienced love through the lens of her reality. Her love gave so much more than any of us could have felt if it weren't for Willow. This was truly an experience that is hard to explain in words, but hopefully if you just shut your eyes and call out Willow's name, you'll feel her love.

The scene brought tears to my eyes as well as to others'. We saw a gal who was born with a birth defect, and yet she had more confidence and pride as she walked through the lobby than any of us possessed on any given day. She brought an immeasurable amount of joy to all those around her with her sweet and innocent smile.

Upon reflection, I realized that she didn't want to be anyone else but herself, nor was she concerned about a few uniform wrinkles or tailor fit pressed scrubs with a perfect crease. She was totally at peace with the world in her own wonderful shell. What a marvelous gift she gave to everyone. There was so little effort for such a grand impact. Clearly, God was shining through.

Note to self: When I am having a bad hair day, a zit on the end of my nose, or a rip in the seat of my pants caused by the gain of an extra few pounds, I've made a promise to myself to make this a "Willow Wednesday Day" and smile through it all. She was a perfect example of what really matters in life. It's not the window dressing, it's what we give from ourselves that is a game changer of life. Our smiles help soften the pain and suffering of many around us, which is especially prevalent in the hospitals. Helping to brighten the day for others is what God chose for me to do. I call this helping with benefits a real win-win.

Thank you, Willow Wednesday, it was *you* who made a difference that day. You showed me the real purpose of life.

# *WINGS OF TWO ANGELS*

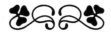

**LIFE IS A** collection of constant journeys. Some are more memorable than others as was this day. When we look outside ourselves and soak in our surroundings, we find the most amazing moments. If we don't look in front and beyond, we miss the stories. This was one of many such journeys that I will hold dear forever.

Volunteering has always been part of my life, but today it took on a new meaning. Little did I know this would be the experience of a lifetime. I volunteered for a group of pilots who donate their private aircrafts and time on a spur-of-the-moment timetable. Collectively, they join together to provide free air transportation for patients in need of medical treatment at distant specialty hospitals. These could be in our state or another state. When asked whether I would assist on one of these flights, my response was an enthusiastic YES! Always fascinated by planes, plus I had taken pilots lessons, so this was a downright awesome offer. No, I was not the pilot. The added bonus for me was that it was a volunteer situation, helping people in need medically and financially by transporting them to a distant hospital for specialized care.

As I was anxiously awaiting the day, it finally arrived. Now, I was standing at the airport next to the pilot and his four-seater plane. It was like a dream. I'm not sure I slept the night before, but as excited as I was, nothing could have prepared me for this moment and the chance of a lifetime. There was nowhere I wanted to be more than right here and now.

There was no audience, no cameras, no applause , no fireworks, or show. The experience was the show. It did not require glitter nor a pep band. This opportunity truly was about to change my life in many ways.

Our mission: flying two small frail patients to a medical center that specialized in a specific research childhood treatment.

"On a wing and a prayer" was a perfect caption for this mission. All other treatment options had not shown any remission of their illness. This was truly a mission of hope.

The skies were thick with an eerie dense fog, lightning ,and intense rain. It was now 5:00 p.m. as we stood at the airport watching a storm as it hovered as if paralyzed over a four-county area, the precise path that was essential for us to fly through. We waited patiently, yet all the while encouraging the storms to move out over the Gulf and beyond. As we tracked every map in every direction, every one indicated the storms were in no hurry to depart.

As we continued observing the weather for optional paths, our passengers arrived at the airport. Two airport stewards approached the plane each carrying a car seats, luggage, formula, and a large box of medicines. A few steps behind, we noted a person that undoubtedly was the very weary young mom. She was barely able to garner enough energy to put one foot in front of the other to walk. These horrific events in life had sucked out every last drop of her energy. We were emotionally focused on the devastating vision of a young woman who not only carried the burden of one child with a terminal illness but also the twin sister. She was holding one of the twins tightly next to her body.

Then we noted a devoted friend walking beside her, carrying the other twin. Both adults were long past complete fatigue.

These precious twins had a fatal childhood disease called congenital lactic acidosis. Almost four years old and weighing shy of 21 lbs. This research program was their last hope. The girls were thin and had sunken dull eyes. Additionally, the mom's eyes were covered with a cataract-like coat of pain, dull and weary. As she handed us her most precious cargo of life, the twins, I fought back my tears. The mother walked back toward the terminal, but her head was looking back and waving while she blew kisses. I told the kids, "Mom is throwing you kisses; see if you can catch them." They mimicked a mumbled giggle, but their little eyes were so heavy that they leaned into their car seats and unsuccessfully fought sleep. Then, I did let my tears flood my face. Even as I write this, the memory is so vivid I relive it each time I think of them. "Our precious angels."

At 6:15 p.m. we got an "all clear" for departure. The words "all clear" did not describe the skies even at the altitude to which we ascended. The twins were awakened with the bumpy air at takeoff but just looked around and fell asleep again.

The saying "In the cool of the evening" did not pertain to this evening. The heat was held down by the dense fog. Our instrument panel registered a hot 85-degree night. The cabin was cooling down with the A/C shortly after liftoff.

It was impossible to not look at the girls. If I looked at them, they would be safe, or so I comforted myself in thinking it so. I quietly sang them a little soft song, which seemed to please them. When my kids were there age, I would do the same. The songs were always made up to fit the situation. This song was about two little angels, flying with the stars, and going to a place where they would meet some new friends. One little angel reached her hand over to her sister and gently placed it onto her arm. Together they fell fast asleep again.

The rest of the flight we heard nary a peep from these two angels. The bumpy ride was no competition in an effort to awaken them.

Upon arrival to our destination, I lifted the two fragile tykes, one by one, from their seats. They were so adorable as they were wearing crisp little white sun dresses and had freshly washed hair, all of which could not mask the aroma of the medicine that permeated their skin—a constant reminder of their struggles until this new effort to reverse their disease course. We entered the hospital lobby, and I leaned down to kiss the neck folds of the twin that I was carrying, and in return, her gift to me, was in showing me a hint of a smile. Without a word, her eyes told me she was not afraid and she was going to be a trooper. I told them, "There are a lot of friends here that will be taking care of you so you both can get well. Watch out for the cute doctors; they like to tickle the kids or so I am told. Always remember, you are not alone. " Her eyes replied in infantile faith, "I know."

This was a first trip of many for the twins and mother. However, it was only the beginning but not an end.

Returning home for us was quiet and reflective. What was there to say? We were reflecting on our part in this mission and hoping we helped get these beautiful and precious girls to received the treatment that was an experiment drug and hopefully would heal them. The pilot and I each knew what the other one of us was feeling and thinking. Silence spoke loudly, and we exchanged an occasional glance followed by a forced smile. The flight home was smooth and swift with the help of a tail wind. The strobe lights, one on each wing, bounced off the clouds like twinkly stars reflecting a glimmer of hope for our precious angels. Their lives depend on the efforts of countless people. Plus lots of prayers and love for the mother too. Special note: pilots and caretakers cry too.

This moment in life touched me to my core. Being able to cradle in my arms these little ones in need, to smell their freshly cleaned skin, to look into their little eyes filled with hope reminds me of how fragile life is and how much we depend on each other. This was the most amazing volunteer job ever.

# ONE OF OUR OWN

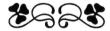

**NURSES ARE THOUGHT** of as personally immune to life's health issues. We do not have time to take off to be sick. We have all the answers on how to fix or prevent anything and everything. After all, we are there to help cure, take care of, and put a special medicated magic Band-Aid on any and every boo-boo that walks, or is wheeled in our door. Rarely, thank goodness, do nurses call off sick. It is an unspoken no-no. A nurse code, so to speak. If someone does call off sick, well, you guessed it, those patients are given to the remaining team. Then to compound the situation, seems as if it is always on a day of having limited staffing and a higher than normal ratio of complicated patients. We anticipate having patients that require more care and attention or a disgruntled family member. But there are those days, sort of like supply and demand, more critical ones to make our teams what we call, "a heavy team." Being in the hospital is a time of stress for not only the patient but the families. Time, money, inconveniences, anxiety, childcare, out of town, and the list of stressors go on and on.

Then the unthinkable happened. A fellow nurse became suddenly ill. Not only a nurse but one with a charge/supervisory position. She was seasoned but young in age and experienced as a manager. It struck the team not only emotionally but physically.

We can't help worry about our "now patient" coworker who is family to each one of us.

Miss "one of us" came from another country alone and without any family to join our hospital team. What a blessing she was. Full of kindness, experience, and talent all in one cute little package. The entire team relied on her wisdom and ability. She was always fair with us and stood ready to roll up her sleeves if needed. On occasion, she would have to give us a tough team on a given day already filled with huge demands, and we would respond with a thank-you. Now that's a great supervisor. She took the term "team" literally. Through her great example, the rest of the team did as well.

News of her health traumatized us all, almost as much as it did her. She was diagnosed with terminal cancer. The worst news, it was rapid growing and her life span would be dramatically shortened, with an expected survival not of years or months, but days, most likely. The doctors left little hope of her leaving the hospital. The most shocking thing was that she never appeared sick. She worked two-day shifts until this day. She was on day three of 12 hrs./day shifts.

While she was in the hospital I talked with her on the phone a few times but could not summon up the courage to physically see her. A coworker stopped me on the way out of work at 8 p.m. that day and said our nurse had taken a turn for the worse. I was only four rooms away from her room. I no longer could put myself first; I told myself that I had to think of her. There was nothing I could do but go into her room. Seeing her in her condition and one of our own were thoughts that kept swirling around in my head. There was only one thing that "turn for the worst" could mean. It was basically imminent.

As I approached her room, the curtains were closed, so the room was dark. She was on isolation. I stood there for a few minutes trying to imagine being in a country with no family and never being able to visit her country and people there ever again. Her family was a 14-hour plane ride away, and it was costly to travel that far, as well. I thought of how awful it would be to die alone when there were plenty of us right there, outside of her room. My decision was, if she could face this horrendous situation, certainly I could show her some love and that she is not alone. I was probably the oldest nurse on the unit, as well as a motherly type. There was absolutely nothing I could reason with that would give me permission to ignore this child lying in there, alone and afraid. I've worked at a trauma hospital, so I've seen things that are difficult to see, but this, it was different. She was a dear hospital staff family member. How could I think I could ignore this? I scolded myself for being afraid to go in to see her. People know me as strong, but this was hard. Afterward, I was glad I went in, and I know she was as well.

I totally disregarded the isolation notice and walked into the silent room. As I quietly walked over to bedside, she looked at me with eyes filled deep with sorrow and pleaded, "They have the wrong reports, these are not my labs and tests, please tell them." I promised her I would.

Then the only thing I could do was to crawl in bed with her and hold her tightly like a child. I was hoping that if I held her tight enough, heaven would wait. All the time I was stroking her hair and telling her all the great things she means to us. I assured her she was strong and she has the best doctors and told her she would beat this thing. Nothing was further from the truth. After she fell asleep, I prayed for about half an hour, begging for her life. Quietly, I slipped out of bed knowing this was my last time with her. As I walked to the door, I looked back at her one last time. "God, be kind with her and give her peace" were the last words I spoke to her.

She is now at peace but not forgotten. She was one of our own who stands as a constant reminder on how rough it is to be a family member with someone you love so dearly in the hospital. I pledged to be more considerate of our patients' family members. Many times I have thought of her as I witnessed families feeling what we all did in our moment of grief.

ONE OF OUR OWN
WE MISS YOU AND LOVE YOU
REST IN PEACE
HEAVEN IS LUCKY

# THE TOUCH OF AN ANGEL WING

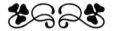

**MY NEW PATIENT** had a stroke a couple days ago and had not yet awakened to voices or stimulation. She was a patient in one of our largest rooms on the unit. As I opened the door, I realized why there was a need for a room this size. Although I didn't count the exact number of her family members and friends that were visiting, I do know it was a lot. They all were seated in chairs and couches that surrounded the room. Later I was informed that the maintenance crew brought in two extra sofas to accommodate them all. Every one of her visitors had a smile. Before entering the room, I heard them singing beautiful hymns. Then standing in the middle of this crowded room, I told them, "The choir was beautiful" and asked them to, "come sing for me if I ever get sick;" their laughter was exceptionally sweet. It was refreshing to see such positive support.

As I turned toward the patient and on my first step toward the bed, I felt a warm gentle breeze on my left shoulder and was brushed with something soft as a feather. I blurted out, "An angel wing just touched my shoulder." Instantly, I was confounded and slightly embarrassed by the words that came out of my mouth. I wasn't sure what to do or say next. The crowded room fell silent. I ignored my outburst and hoped they did too. Truly, I didn't know what happened or how to explain my outburst, so I just walked to the patient's bedside and proceeded to examine her. The minute I laid my stethoscope on her, she instantly opened her eyes and smiled at me. I was as shocked as her visitors were. Chills ran up and down my spine. I had taken care of many stroke patients and saw them as they recovered from a stroke, but this was so spontaneous it felt as though we had just witnessed a miracle. I was certainly a believer that day.

It is not unusual for a stroke patient to wake out of their comma, but it was the most amazing thing I have ever seen or felt. Turning toward the friends and family, I said, "Your words of prayer and songs of joy invited an angel to come in. God has given you your wishes, and he hears you all. I'm sure none of us will ever forget this. Thank you for letting me be here with you all. You'll have to tell Mom what happened here today. Enjoy your blessed day." With that, I turned and left the room, but a piece of her will always remain in my heart.

The room instantly filled with a big celebration highlighted with more songs, clapping to the beat of gospel music. It felt as though Sunday services came to the hospital that day. I did not tell the patient what happened, I left that for the family to share. I hardly believed it, but it was real. I'll never forget that brush on my shoulder.

Each one thanked me, but I reminded them it wasn't me. It was their vigil and hope that brought the angel. We all witnessed that they do exist.

# *THE CARROT CAKE WEDDING*

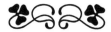

**MY DAY STARTED** like all others with a report from the night nurse about the patients that had been assigned to me. I reviewed my patients meds, labs, timelines, and procedures along with their level of care and special needs. This helped me be prepared for possible surprises that might and more often do happen. My to-do list involves an hour-by-hour must-do responsibilities. Every one of us has our own way to approach the day what works for them.

My first patient, was room 305: poor prognosis, vent, tube feed, terminal lung cancer. My most critical patient. I decided to see him first and confirm that my plans matched his needs for the day.

Being respectfully quiet, I greeted him with a soft, "How are you doing this morning?" What came next were snapshots of a patient that didn't look like the picture that the night nurse described to me or the reflections of his chart.

"I'm fabulous," the patient stated with a strong convincing voice.

"What makes you fabulous today?" I said.

"I'm getting married today," the patient replied.

I was trying to assess a patient who was not exhibiting the clinical picture represented in the chart, nor in the morning report. I felt like my first day in nursing. What was I missing here? He was on a vent, unable to get out of bed and a hundred other reasons that I personally would not consider as being fabulous. Then, getting married? Sounded like a man that was delusional.

So I continued to investigate and question further. "That's nice. Tell me about it," I queried.

With more energy than I had, he proceeded to tell me about this wonderful woman who he has lived with for 13 years, the love of his life. He assured me his brother got the marriage license, then he went to pick up the unsuspecting bride-to-be to bring her to the hospital. She didn't know they were going to get married today.

Now, I was really confused.

"I'm going to get married right here in his room," my patient stated.

Of course, his story did not end here. The bride was totally unaware of his plans. "We talked about it before but never got married. Things always got in the way, and we eventually said we are happy and don't need to get married. I figured now is the time. I want to show her how much I love her," he added.

Oh boy, this could end well or not. I chose to believe this would go well and that the rest of my patients were not planning any such major events for the day.

All my planning, prioritizing, stick to the plan attitude, and the gaps left open for minor surprises certainly did not factor his enormous plans into my schedule.

Within a few short moments, here was his brother and the unknowing bride coming down the hall for what she assumed was only a much-anticipated visit. She walked into the room, and after maneuvering around the equipment, she gave him a sweet hug and kiss. Then, I heard her scream, "YES." I knew I had to make this work. Oh my gosh, this is really happening. I think I was as surprised as she was. And strangely enough, almost as excited.

Quickly, I rallied the staff around to explain the situation and solicit a team effort to care for the other patients. After they looked at me like I was crazy, they were all in. The longer they thought about it, the more excited everyone was.

First and foremost, I couldn't let them get married in a dark dreary room. This is going to be a challenge with all the required equipment pumping and hissing and a frame hovering over him like an erector set attached to the bed. My first words darted out like an army sergeant commanding his new recruits. "You can't get married in the room," I said sternly. The shocked looks and disappointment was written all over their faces. I feel they thought this was a statement as if the hospital was forbidding it. With a softer voice and some further explanation, their expressions changed into a more relaxed look.

I want to be your wedding planner. Wow, now I have shocked them again. Puzzled looks returned to their faces. I assured them it will all work out and we will make it special. I promised.

Without a plan in place yet my unvalidated certainty made me a bit concerned. I needed to get hospital clearance. Oops. It's like doing the surgery but forgetting to fill out the forms and get a signature. But "I promised" were words that swirled around in my head. I was about to be in deep do-do. Not a first for me I assure you.

Then arose, and my inner muse, who gets me in trouble a lot, poked me to say to the couple, "The chapel is available, and I'm going to figure out a way to make this memorable." Tears erupted from their eyes as she said, "That would be amazing." Just seeing her excitement, I continued to promise more by saying, "Let me work on that, and you two just dream together." There I went with more words uttered while floating in this dream world of promises I was part of. Let me correct that, I was the instigator, not just a part of. I was willing to take any and all responsibility. Too late to back out now.

I kicked up my responsibilities of being a nurse to three other patients. Every patient's medications were pulled, I reviewed their vitals, prepared discharge orders for two patients, and proceeded to their rooms, one by one. I approached every patient with my normal exam and explanations of their care plan for the day. Also asked them if that had anything special they needed that I could get them. I breathed a big sigh of relief when every single one of them said they didn't need anything.

Before I left each room, I explained that something special was happening today and I would like to make them a part of it. "We have never done this before, to my knowledge, but one of our patients is getting married," I said with exaggerated enthusiasm. I further explained the couple's situation, for which I had gotten permission from them to share their story. I told them that when they come up from the chapel we would like them to be standing in their doorway to cheer for the new husband and wife. No one refused. In fact, the excitement was wild with cheers and positive feedback on how the hospital was supporting this.The immediate Kudos for the hospital were all extremely positive.

Now I was committed, and I probably should have been committed in another way too. Sometimes I need to learn to just step aside. But the looks on the faces of everyone were priceless. At least I choose to interpret it that way. Nothing worse than a crazy nurse, right?

I told the couple how exciting this is and how much the patients would love to share in the joy.

Luckily, my other patients required a low level of monitoring, and a couple were slated for probable discharge when the doctors make rounds, thus requiring little attention. After I attended to these patients and informed them of all the plans for this wedding, they were so excited that I really didn't hear a peep out of them. But they were not ignored, regardless. I did notice that I didn't have to tell them to get out of bed and walk a little, either.

Then came a parade of patients and family walking circles around the nurses' station. Lots of thumbs-up, smiles, and OK gestures were given by the staff. The entire department shared in all the duties of patient care and planning needs. Kudos to an amazing hospital and its staff! The team was fabulous as always.

I did call management to get approval (a little later than I should have, but I said a prayer before asking and after just to cover my bases with God). With their blessing I began to scheme even bigger. Chapel and chaplain were on board with the idea (plus the chaplain gave the couple a Bible).

Respiratory Dept.: agreed to free up staff to transport the patient to the chapel and back (staying with them the entire time). This was an amazing gesture, which they executed perfectly and professionally. Note: it took four people to safely transport the bed and equipment to the chapel.

Gift Shop: arranged a bridal bouquet of a large white lily in full bloom with the yellow stamen shining bright and happy like a ray of sunshine. Upon entering the chapel, we were again met with a vision of love. Celebration also followed them into the chapel with an array of white/silver balloons.

Nurses, techs, and the secretary all made confetti out of the printer paper, and we made a door sign saying, "Congratulations Mr. and Mrs.," which was posted to the door with scotch tape.

The administration arranged for pictures to be taken by our marketing staff.

The cafeteria said they could provide cake to share with the entire floor/patients, family, and visitors, too.

Now, all the plans were set in motion, and all within three hours. In my mind I rationalized that life gives us moments where we have to step forward and uplift others in need. It is an obligation, in a world where serious situations fall unexpectedly upon people to lend a hand of compassion. She deserved a wedding as beautiful as she was.

# THE WEDDING

**THE BRIDE WAS** given her beautiful bouquet made from a white lily and green vining sprays trailing down over her hands. The groom had a white rose pinned to his hospital gown. Somehow, it didn't seem odd; it was beautiful.

The Respiratory Dept. wheeled him in his bed, along with his vent and other equipment in tow, to the chapel. His bride walked by his side holding hands as they gazed at each other in a way that would melt anyone's heart. He looked at her and said, "You are truly beautiful." A little piece of tulle gathered together with a pink ribbon and a white rose was pinned to her hair, another donation by the gift shop. She truly look like a bride and was simply beautiful.

Our chaplain proceeded to give a personalized wedding vow service. Adding to the special event was a gal that plays a harp in our main lobby. She came to the chapel to offer a few heavenly tunes.

The Respiratory Dept. notified us that they were on their way back to the room. The door frame around his room was covered with white and silver balloons, a "MR & MRS" hand-drawn sign was taped to the door, and the other patients were standing in their doorways waiting for the new couple to arrive. When the couple turned the corner to enter the main area known as the nurses' station, everyone erupted in applause and cheers. We carefully tossed our homemade confetti, light bulbs flashed, and the chaplain had a beautiful wedding song playing on a recorder.

Soon he was all settled into his room with all of his equipment properly working. I checked on him to verify he was not in any distress from the travel and excitement. His smile told me the whole story.

Without any delay, the kitchen was rolling a cart loaded with wedding cake slices. With the nurse's approval, patients and anyone who walked by, were given a piece of wedding cake. People came from other floors as well just to see what was going on.

It was not a typical wedding. But it could not have been any better. The cake was special as well. It was a carrot cake. We wouldn't have had it any other way. It was a special cake for a very special day. The chef apologized, but that was all he had in the freezer. I turned toward the crowd, all eating the cake, and said, "Who's glad this wedding cake is a carrot cake and not a white cake?" Again, cheer filled the room. The cake was a big hit. Memories were being made, and this was certainly one of the highlights.

My biggest thank you goes to our Respiratory Department. They did all the work and this couldn't have happened without them. Our HEROS for sure.

A thank-you goes out the cleaning staff who cleaned up the confetti mess. For heaven's sake the confetti was everywhere. Kudos to the Respiratory Dept. Not a one of them complained. They were just glad to be part of the celebration, plus they got some cake. We only saw smiles among us all.

As the bride left to go home, she went to all the doors and nurses' station and thanked everyone for the most memorable day of her life. She said she will never forget each and every one. Her tears of joy were confirmation that this was the biggest gift we could give them. I told her she will be long remembered and the patients felt the same.

When we compared notes at the end of the day, we realized every single patient was happy and excited the entire day. They all thought this was the most amazing gift from the staff they have ever seen in a hospital. My response was, "We care above and beyond in this hospital." It made the day for the couple, the patients, and the staff.

Now that's a day in the life of a nurse. Every day provides different challenges, joy, sorrow, love, creative thinking, and devotion. They aren't all tough days. The good days and amazing patients help us feel rewarded more than can be measured.

Sadness doesn't always have to overshadow the joys in life. Today was a great example and validated by the bride as she exclaimed, "This is the best day of my life". We couldn't change the inevitable, but we gave them a wedding that was a celebration greater than any they could have imagined.

Last, but not least, thank you to the Hospital Administration for having a belief in all of us to make this a positive day for everyone. The go ahead we were given made a very special couple's wish come true. There were things we could not cure but we found a dream we could give.

# THE ROSARY

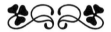

**EVERY PATIENT IS** like a new story. But to a nurse, we enter a room on Chapter 10, with no Cliff Notes. We know very well what the medical needs of the patient are and have a very well-thought-out plan of care. Knowing the patient is a very different thing for each one.

I knew that Maria was terminally ill and had just prior to my entering the room, been delivered the news from her doctor that they have exhausted every lifesaving option possible. This is the kind of morning you wished the doctor had not shown up early. Or shall I say, just right before you entered the room. A flood of thoughts circled in my head: "Was she alone, was she distraught, was she angry, was she uncontrollably crying, is there family there," only to mention a few possible options.

"Hello, Maria, my name is Pam. I'm going to be your nurse today." That was about as generic as I could be. I couldn't have anticipated what the next two days would bring. Maria had a warm smile that felt inviting. She felt like a mother who was saying, "Come on in now and sit down. Have something to eat." Spanish-speaking with just a little, very little English. So I thought, my first challenge was communication. She reached out to take my hand and kissed the top. I thought, "Whew, good start."

I learned quickly that Maria had a very deep faith and that the rosary was always clutched in her hand. We had worked out a way to talk through sign language (made up signs) and motions and mannerisms. She told me how she went to Italy and the rosary was blessed by the pope. This was her most treasured possession. Every morning and night with hands that felt like velvet, she gently placed the rosary between my hand and hers. She prayed over our hands. Even with a language challenge, I understood her well as she did me. She was so cute that If I didn't understand her, she would reach up and touch my cheek, shake her head, and smile. We both would laugh. It was with kindness and caring that I would also hold her face in my hands. What an amazing woman. Her deep faith transcended words. There wasn't anything forced in her faith, it was real and Heaven-sent for sure.

What an amazing spirit she had. Her room was always calm, peaceful, content, inviting, and a refuge from the hustle and bustle of my job. Here was a patient that was taking care of me and making me the focus of love and care. Two days was all I was blessed to spend with her. At the end of each day, we would each say a prayer with our hands coupled together with her rosary as our bond of faith in-between. I would kiss her on the forehead and said, "Mañana," exercising my "extensive" Spanish vocabulary. I'm letting you know that my Spanish vocabulary has increased to 25 words currently.

The following day, just before the end of my shift, she was transferred from our critical care floor to a medical floor. I remember walking along side of her gurney to the elevator. Once again Maria took my hand just before the elevator doors opened. She placed her rosary in my hand and in very plain English said, "God told me he wanted you to have this." With obvious tears in my eyes, I told her I wasn't allowed to accept gifts, but she said, "a Gift from God." As the tears streamed down my face, she looked at me and smiled and said, "Gracias" while blowing me a kiss. She didn't shed a tear; her eyes were dry and loving. The smile on her face was confirmation of total contentment. Her faith had brought her through life, and now she accepted her next journey with grace. After being wheeled into the elevator, the doors closed. I kept watching her through the crack of the two doors until they were closed tightly. Desperately, I wanted to pry the doors open and refuse to let her go.

It wasn't a work day, but I went to see Maria the next morning. As I passed the nursing station, the charge nurse called me over to the desk. She wanted to tell me Maria passed last night in her sleep. It was just like Maria to do that. She fell asleep peacefully. I choose to remember holding her hands, so full of love and happiness. She would not want me to remember her by how painful it was to see those elevator doors close. I accepted her loving glow and will try to generate the same trust she had to the very end.

For the next 20+ years, I carried that rosary with me to work every day. Since I've retired from nursing, I keep the rosary in a heart-shaped bone china dish beside my bed. I've held that rosary several times and thought of her and prayed for God to give me half of the ability to care for others as she shared with me. I know she is touching my cheek, and I saw her smiling at me every time I held her rosary in my hand. Maria lives on in my heart and in my caring for others. Maria, I hope you approve.

Maria, I will pass this Rosary onto my nurse someday when I make the journey as well.

# *LAUGHTER IS THE BEST MEDICINE*

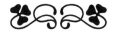

**THE UNIQUENESS OF** every patient is what makes a nurse's job challenging and interesting. It's like watching 5 TV shows at once. Every show has a different plot and we strive to keep up with the characters while fulfilling our role.

Mr. Jones was not what I would expect from a stroke patient. He was sitting up in the recliner beside his bed and smiling as I walked into his room. I began the normal introduction and questioning on how he was doing, and an explanation of what the plans were for the day.

In walks our Occupational Therapist (OT) with her list of activities as well for his therapy for today. It was clear the two of us have planned a very busy day for him.

Mr. Jones started joking around and the two of us fed into his humor quickly. We were all loving every moment of this banter. The saying, "Laughter Is The Best Therapy ", is very true. However, I believe the doctors and pharmacists would take exception to this remark.

Being a patient provides very little material for laughter. Unless you are Mr. Jones. In any case this would not be considered a trip to the amusement park. First thing, we take this guy and make him suffer the indignity of wearing a hospital gown. Let's call it what it is, a dress with a draft. A vivid picture, right?

Additionally, every professional that walks into his room would do a thorough exam and ask every personal question imaginable. I'm sure the patient is thinking, why don't you read the chart buddy. Then, just as you think you have stripped the patient of all self respect and privacy, we parade him around the halls in the latest style dress/gown with a gap of 6" or more down the back. Thus, relieving him of any missed thread of dignity that my be left or missed. Who knows, the last 15 people that have visited him with their list of questions may have missed something.

Only Mr. Jones could see the humor in this. His jokes were better than any stand up comedy routine. We provided him with the perfect audience. US, the OT and myself. We were starved for a little bit of levity in our serious work day.

During one of our many silly times, I told him the OT was my daughter. I told him this after he was telling her how pretty and sweet she was. His first reaction was, "No, you're messing with me". My convincing skills even exceeded my normal abilities that day. He bought into the notion that she really was my daughter. We did have some features that could be claimed as family features. However she was young, thin, blonde, and sweet. I'm not positive those traits and qualities totally represented myself. Maybe my blonde highlights made it believable. But, we went with it and he was sold our bill of goods. In retrospect, we should have raised the stakes given he bought into our scam so quickly.

Just because we laughed and enjoyed each other didn't indicate his care was neglected. He wholeheartedly participated in his therapy. Like a child or father, he didn't want to disappoint us.

It was day 3 and we were both in his room on our final rounds for the day when his wife walked in. "So you are the two my hubby tells me about", she said. Oh boy, my mind was racing and hoping this was a good thing. Then smiling she told us, "He said you two were so much fun and even what was better was that you are mother and daughter." With a face that represented a poster of a criminal, I confessed, "Well, I lied. But perhaps you can forgive me if I amend that and say, Hospital Mother and Daughter".

This family was the cherry on top of the sundae for the both of us. He was compliant and respected our roles while adding some grumpy ole man humor to make us laugh. But our fun was coming to a close as it was discharge day. It will feel strange not to have him in that room. But, we did our jobs and he was ready for discharge. He confessed the only thing he would miss was us.

His lovely wife was walking him out after being given his discharge papers and I of course couldn't let him go without one more spark of humor. I called down the hall and said, "Come Back Soon". He laughed one last time and said, "I love you two". We both blew him a kiss.

# NINE LANGUAGES

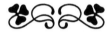

**ROOM 1317 WAS** quiet and dark. In bed lay a small lady, about four feet ten, fast asleep. On the whiteboard I wrote my name, date, day of the week, and drew a flower in the corner of the board, the one thing and only thing I could draw. I walked quietly to give the patient time to gently wake up. I pulled the curtain separating the unoccupied bed between her and the door. I turned on the light over the vacant bed. While replacing a bag of fluids, I started softly humming/singing "Amazing Grace." Guess it came to my mind as her name was Grace. It was in a whispered singing voice, one that you can't tell whether the person has a voice or not.

During this morning's nursing report I had been informed that the patient was nonverbal for the past 24 hours. So I was totally and pleasantly surprised when the patient said in broken English, "I love music." And then, before I could introduce who I was, she proceeded to tell me she sings in nine languages. "I don't know what the words mean but as a child listened to radio and learned the songs." My assessment went from nonverbal to chatty. Note: I had little air time; she was quite the character.

Then the routine started, and the lights came on over her bed, allowing me to properly assess this not so nonverbal patient.

After my morning assessment, I walked back to the white-board and wrote the numbers one through nine. "Miss Grace," I said, "I'm going to be in here nine times today to hear you sing to me, and I'll write the language after each number."

She was thrilled knowing I'd visit that many times and that she could share her talent. Before I left her room I said, "Oh, by the way, my name is Pam and I'm your nurse. I love to sing but frequently am told not to. So I look forward to your voice".

I would walk into the room and act like a radio announcer. "Audience, Here's Ms. Grace to sing you another wonderful song. She hails from Scotland but has been touring throughout Europe this past year. Hopefully, she will be coming to your town soon." I'd announce, "Song number six," or whatever number we were on. "The phone lines are busy, but please be patient. Keep your requests coming. Ms. Grace, please tell us the language you are going to sing for us now." She would tell me, and I would fill in the language on the next blank on the board.

When she got to number nine, I teased her about exaggerating and really only knowing eight languages, reminding her that she could only win the grand prize if she completed all nine languages. What a laugh we had. However, she did not disappoint: all nine languages were confirmed.

I learned early on that every patient has a uniqueness. When we figure out how to tap that special something, they become easier to understand, and they become more comfortable in expressing their feelings and symptoms. I like leaving them with a trust knowing that I will take care of them. For Ms. Grace, she was able to open up with the doctors. They were able to treat her and discharged her the next day.

I wasn't there, but I'll bet she was singing all the way down the hall when she was going home. I'm just not sure, but perhaps it was language #10, one she forgot to tell me about.

Keep Singing.

# HIDDEN PAIN

**ROSIE, A 45** year old female was very quiet and soft spoken patient. She didn't have any visitors the past 3 days while I was her nurse except at 6PM when her husband would show up for about an hour. She was admitted for intestinal pain and severe reflux. Diagnostic tests indicated esophageal ulcers from acid reflux. Additionally she had a fairly elevated blood pressure that is now being successfully treated with medications. In addition to her reflux meds, she was medically ready for discharge.

Day 2 of her stay, Rosie began to smile and was more open to conversation than her first day on our unit. I credited this to her new medications. We discussed some proper diet changes and options that would help reduce and hopefully avoid the onset recurrence of the reflux.

Day 3, the doctor prepared her discharge and follow up orders. He recommended an appointment with a GI Physician as well as a Cardiologist. I told her I had the discharge paperwork but could delay them until her husband could pick her up at his normal 6:00 pm.

She told me she still did not feel well enough and would like to stay and have these doctors see her while she was in the hospital. I explained to her that she only needs to see them as an outpatient and as a follow up for her new medications.

About 1PM I went into her room with her paperwork for discharge. She was extremely nervous and fidgety. This was a dramatic change from anything I saw from her since admission. I asked if she was OK and she looked down and in a sad voice said, "I'll be ok." But within a few moments she began to weep uncontrollably. We talked a little while in order to let her settle down before I started digging into the real reasons for all these abrupt emotional bursts during discharge.

"Are you afraid to go home", I asked bluntly? Without hesitation she said, "Petrified". I left the room for a moment and called a social worker.

When I came back to her room, she pleaded with me not to let her husband know she told me that she was afraid. "He drinks a lot and gets really mad at me whatever I say and he punches me in my stomach and shoves me." She unleashed her tale of horrific abuse and continued fears as her voice quivered.

We moved her to another room on another floor and assigned her an assumed name immediately. It was discovered that the police had been called to their home on numerous occasions and she had a broken bone in her neck and arm and wrist. Her X-rays confirmed that she has had a history of multiple fractures.

After discharge, she was moved to a safe house and given an opportunity to start a new life.

There are way too many of these abusive scenarios. Only a small portion are ever reported. Fear allows us to accept abuse while shame allows us to hide the humiliating facts while showing how weak the victims are. They find themselves living in a bubble of shame and fear.

I was glad to have helped one of these victims and hopefully, we as healthcare workers, can continue to identify and save others.

# *COVID-19 VACCINATIONS*

**CAN YOU IMAGINE** how giving a vaccination can bring joy to the day? Well, here's how it did for me and the lovely lady I was fortunate enough to meet.

Our hospital vaccination clinic was set up in one of our remote hospitals, and I volunteered to work two 12-hour shifts that week. The people who came for their vaccines were full of all kinds of stories. I think the anxiety made them more talkative as a distraction from the long needle I was about to poke them with. A majority of them were from a nearby retirement housing development. I tried to hide a glimpse of the needle from them but wasn't always successful. However, I did manage to insert the needle while we were talking. Typically the patients hardly realized I had given them the vaccine until I put a Band-Aid over it. Distraction is the greatest nursing tool. Well, maybe not the greatest, but it is right up there.

My most memorable patient was a little elderly woman. She was well manicured and polite but seemed to have a sadness about her. Initially, we exchanged very few words except for my instructions. As I reached out to support her elbow while trying to help her remove her coat, she began to tear up. Instantly, I feared somehow her arm was tender and I had moved it in a painful way. I apologized for hurting her. "No, thank you," she said, which was a response I imagined was for my apology. Rather, she told me her husband passed away in August, a few months earlier, and that is the first time someone has touched her since then. I took both of her hands while looking into her eyes, and told her, "He touches your heart each day, and I hope you remember that." She reached up and put a hand on each of my cheeks and said, "Bless you." In response, I let her know that she had already blessed me just by being here. I said to her, "The good memories were meant to be cherished. Laugh at the silly times. Talk to him out loud. Scold him for leaving you, but remind him you will be there some day and remind him how much it hurt to let him go."

She never felt the vaccine.

This is what nursing is all about. I am so glad I got to be there. As nurses, we give more than we think, and we get much more than we realize. I know, I've kept track.

# HEART TRANSPLANT/
# MOTHER OF TWO

**IT IS ONLY** natural to have an emotional attachment to your patients. Even the ones that give you a challenge. Being seriously ill can complicate and escalate human reactions to the known and unknown parts of treatments.

I worked with a heart transplant team while loving most of the highly sensitive and fast pace challenges. The team of physicians were highly vetted making every day another string of invaluable lessons. It would take years to learn what they taught me in months. This staff of physicians were aligned with an educational program and they treated me like one of their budding students. I of course was not a physician, nor was I a student in medical school, nor was I a nurse with 20 years experience. But, I was 40 years plus in age and I imagine they considered me a seasoned nurse do to my age. I never tried to correct them on their impression.

After leaving work at night, I would go to the medical library and review patient's procedures and diagnosis' from the day and study their medications. I learned as much as I could about the equipment and the new upcoming medical treatments. I tried never to ask a question I hadn't already done my homework on. I wanted to ask intelligent questions. Then I would have a basic understanding and their answers made sense. I was single and since this was my income, I wanted to be the best that I could be.

The doctors would see me in the library and smile but never disturbed me. I think they were impressed, which was not my purpose. I just wanted to know what I was doing. They had no idea how basic my knowledge was. Every hour of study was well worth it and within a couple months, I really did feel like I fit in. Not to the physician level but enough to know who to ask if I didn't know or understand. Every one of them was more than willing to answer any questions I had. Studying before asking helped me look better. What an amazing group of physicians. I coined them my walking encyclopedias.

We admitted patients who were in heart failure and required the use of an external machine that basically acted as a temporary heart pump (replaces the job of a patient's heart when it fails). The patients are placed on this until a donor match can be found. This was not a permanent fix machine but kept the patient alive until a donor heart can take its place. During the time I worked in this department, these machines were about the size of the carts the airline attendants would push down the aisle to serve beverages. BIG in other words. Within a year and a half they evolved into a portable, to keep my description simple, the size of a buddy waist pack and shoulder straps.

One of my precious patient's was a young mother of 2 pre-school children. The vision of the perfect couple, kids, and life. However, it wasn't what the medical team would call her condition. She was diagnosed with Heart Failure right after her second child was born. She was put on our Left Ventricular Assist machine and put high priority on the heart transplant list for a donor.

The brother and baby sister loved snuggling with mom and the son occasionally used the bed as a trampoline. Mom and Dad tried to keep things as normal as they could while going through the toughest time of their lives.

A match was found. The moment the heart was delivered to the Operating Room, she was wheeled into surgery. The couple was so excited and ready to move on with their lives and raising these two little munchkins.

The moment she was wheeled back into her room for recovery, there was her smiling husband. He looked 10 years younger than before, to me. Stress can do that. What a moment of true celebration. Grandma had the kids but would bring them as soon as it was cleared by the doctor.

On Day 3 after the implant, I went in to her room where she and her husband were relaxing and enjoying the peace and quiet.

As I was speaking to the patient, without warning, she looked startled and started gasping for air. I instantly rang the alert call bell and a team of 6 physicians poured into the room. A call for all hands on deck. One of them jumped onto the cart over her trying to pump her heart as they wheeled her back to the OR.

I sat with the husband who was in a full flood stage of tears. I had no answers for him. I had nothing. Waiting seemed like torture. However, in contrast, when you receive bad news, you suddenly wish you could wait a little longer.

The pastor came in and sat with the husband while they awaited the news. Then the doctor came in and told the husband she didn't make it. She had rejected the heart and it failed. Everyone at the nurses station knew by the scream of agony what the answer was. These are the days you wish you weren't on duty and the most horrific days in the doctor's career. But it happens. That doesn't make it any easier though.

I remember walking into my next room after I got the news and it was all I could do to not burst out crying. There was a gentleman, 70 yo laying in his bed and 10 days post transplant. He began scolding me about the staff he called 15 minutes ago for someone to bring him some water. During his visit he was unhappy about everything. I didn't even see the joy that generally comes after a successful heart transplant. If his gift of life can't make him smile, what could?

I often wonder if I could have told him the story of the family in the room down the hall and their loss of a mother, wife, and the immense grief that her children and husband were experiencing, would he then feel blessed to have been given the gift of life or would he jump over their tragic issue and straight back to being cranky for being denied water for 15 min.

Another example that life is not always fair. I hope the family was able to ultimately have some happiness in their lives. I know a beautiful family of two kids and a brave man that do.

# MAY, NOT JUNE

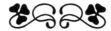

**THE DAY WAS** sunny with a gentle cool breeze making the weather perfect. My job was manager for a nursing staffing agency. We placed nurses and aides into facilities experiencing a long-term or situational, temporary nursing shortage. My first stop was a local and very charming nursing home. My approach to soliciting any staffing was through an in-person visit. This became a very successful approach touch that personally exhibited our company's caring attitude. It was my way of showing this is a "*who* we are," not just "*what* we are" approach. We had an excellent staff available to fulfill multiple support positions for any shortages they might experience. As in any introduction, in person proved to be beneficial. The effort put into showing up as a manager opened many doors. The business was thriving, and I never stopped showing up in person.

As I left the facility, there was this sweet little lady bundled up in a short jacket topped with a stylish pink flowered scarf. A cane leaned against the bench beside her. She sat on the black wrought iron bench with such a proper erect posture with her hands cupped on top of each other and on her lap as though she were waiting for a handsome date to pick her up. Her cute short legs did not touch the ground even as she was sitting toward the edge on the bench. As expected, she was swinging them as she welcomed the sun's warmth. Beside her lay a petite black purse with pink trim matching her pink flowered scarf. It was so adorable, almost as much as she was, but too small to carry any more than a photo ID and lipstick. She had pantyhose on with orthopedic-looking shoes, but they were not boring. In concert with her attire her shoes sported a one-inch heel. Everything supported her readiness to meet whatever or whomever she was waiting for.

One look at her, and I knew her life had a very interesting story. I felt it would be exciting to sit with her awhile if she didn't mind. My thoughts drifted with thoughts of where was she going. She appeared to be going to an event that required a little more attention than everyday clothes.

I started with, "Good morning, my dear. Are you waiting on a bus?" to which she replied, "No, just dreaming." "Well," I said, "every day is a good day to dream, so I'm glad you are. Do you mind if I sit with you and dream as well?" Her smile was as inviting as the sun. "That would be wonderful," she replied.

As I sat beside her, I noted my feet did meet the ground, and I was unable to enjoy the childish joy of swinging my legs, a pleasure she deserved. Expectedly, she introduced herself in such a cute, sparky way, "I'm May, not June, but May". We both giggled as my thoughts raced to the thousands of questions I had while anxiously awaiting our conversation. She had more spunk in her than myself, who was a minimum of 50 years younger. That says a lot as I am not one that lacks conversation or activity.

Her accent initiated my first question. I wanted to know what country she was from. Intently I listened to her life story as she lovingly relived the most cherished tales. Every word she spoke was a vivid recreation of her life. I mentally saw a movie script being created in my mind from her descriptions in such great detail. She made it so interesting, I couldn't bear the thought of having to leave. Her face was like a picture show and displayed her story with an expression that matched the joy all the way to and through her tragic life's events.

She said she was born in a communist country. Then, one day, she and her daughter boarded a ship headed to the United States. Her husband and son stood at the dock watching as they waved goodbye to each other. They would stay behind to run the business. Faithfully, he sent money monthly to the States for their support. Years went by, until the day came she had always feared. The money stopped coming. The war had escalated, and of course she assumed the worse. After numerous and unsuccessful attempts to secure any information on their fate, she learned to accept the probable outcome. Her sad eyes looked into mine as if she could no longer see. She was numb, and the pain of loss was branded deeply into her soul for life. Her eyes revealed an emptiness of loss. Wow, I'm sure she saw the tears that welled up in my eyes. She took my hands and smiled. Following this sorrowful personal flashback in her life, I saw another amazing transformation of joy in her eyes. It was as though she had a light switch that she could turn on and off in order to survive the worst of times and thoughts.

"My husband would want me to live the life he provided for me and not relive the excruciating pain of loss. So that is my focus while mostly embracing the joyful times we had and the times he secured for me to spend with our daughter. All the while he provided well for us, and we lacked for nothing except for him and our son." Her daughter got married to a fine young man, and she too was blessed with a new life in the arms of America. "They would not want us to be sad," she added.

Here was an adorable elderly woman who is still counting her blessings amid extreme life changes and uncertainty. What an example. Maybe that's how she lived to be in her 90s and maintaining a smile.

The initial mission this day was to go to a nursing home and secure a contract. However, each day I find that the road maps and plans in life lead us on detours. This was one detour that was worth every moment and one that continues to bless my life. She continues, long after she is gone, to give goodness.

# A LIGHT THAT STILL
# SHINES—MAY

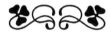

**A FEW YEARS** went by, but I never forgot "May, not June. My thoughts drifted back to her while walking through an arts and crafts store that was going out of business. It was the week after Thanksgiving.

I thought maybe the Christmas section would have some crazy deal I couldn't refuse. Everything was 70 percent off. They had lots of the little Christmas village homes that I loaded up on for Christmas gifts.

Just when I thought I was ready to check out, there stood a shelf full of battery-operated short string lights. Instantly, I thought of "May, not June." There were 15 short strings left on the shelf, and every one of them went into my cart. My thought was instant and unexpected as it had been a few years since I thought of May. May's cane and the bright lights of her charm can shine again today. She had passed away, but her light remained and should be shared.

As I walked into the nursing home, I was hoping my plan would be approved. As usual, I was ahead of my plan and now had to find a way to implement it with the nursing home management.

The manager met me at the desk where my experience and plan was explained. My mission would be to change her look of "I don't think so" to a "yes!" After explaining who May was, my plea jumped right into the convincing story. It would be perfect to give a little Christmas joy and wrap the residents' canes in a string of lights. The manager wasn't convinced, so I stretched my plea further and suggested they play Christmas music in the living room and turn the lights down low. Or maybe I can get a carol group from one of the schools to come sign a couple of songs. Now a smile was coming across her face.

Everyone knows how when you try to convince someone, you keep promising till you see a yes in their eyes. We learn this as a child, don't we?! What got the YES and OK? For those who don't have canes, I plan to bring something to decorate their doors. I even got a, "That sounds nice." With a huge thank-you, I told her I would do all the work and let her know the plans before I move ahead. Whew, my next option would have been Christmas dinner! Not really. I set my limits lower than that.

The results were even better than I could have expected. An elementary group from a church came and sang a few songs. They were positively adorable.

May, thank you for being you. You have brought a story and light from beyond. Heaven is lucky to have you, and so were we. Keep shining your light.

# *"HEY NURSE, I NEED YOU IN HERE"*

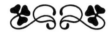

**I WAS IN** the hallway when I heard a doctor urgently holler, "NURSE, I NEED YOU IN HERE." Therefore, into the room I went.

There was an elderly man breathing rapidly while gasping for breath. He was sitting on the side of his bed with his arms stretched over a bedside tray table. The physician was going to perform a Thoracentesis procedure, which is a procedure to aspirate fluid from lungs with a long needle introduced through his back and into his lung. This is a bedside procedure. But with the patient's severe shortness of breath it is very scary to lean over a table enabling him to stretch his back out giving the doctor better access. It is not untypical to be anxious. Anxiety also makes the breathing harder, the combination of which leads to a feeling of panic. Well, this patient was in full-panic mode, which is not the ideal condition in such a procedure.

"I need some help here to keep the patient calm," said the doctor, who was behind the patient. He smiled and added a heartfelt "Please." This was not my patient, but he really did need help, and I appreciated his kind approach.

I said, "Well, Mr. Stanton, your day will soon to be getting better. Once that fluid is gone, you'll be able to take a nice deep breath. No don't forget we don't allow any running down the hallway. The doctor is about to perform a miracle right here in this room." Anyone who knows me, I can talk a person's leg off (pun), and the more I talked, the less he thought about the procedure. I stroked his head, like one would a child sleeping on one's lap, and I held his hands with my other hand. I remember saying, "You know, this table is for eating on, not sleeping on." Then I thought, "Oh boy, please don't laugh, as the doc will shoot me if you move." Instantly wiser, as the doctor was about to begin, I changed my tone to a soft voice and talked to him about my new dog. True confession, I didn't have a new dog. Continuing to talk and holding his hands, he remained perfectly calm, as if he had forgotten the doctor was even there. Mission accomplished. "OK, Mr. Stanton, good job. We got a lot of fluid off, and you should be a lot more comfortable," stated the doctor.

The next day, again I heard someone holler, "Nurse, can you come in here?" The patient was sitting up in bed with a big smile on his face. He said, "I never got to see you, but I knew that was your voice in the hallway. You were here yesterday, right?" to which I confessed. He told me that I was so kind and my voice got him through. He said he would have never made it without me. Maybe that was a stretch, but I chose to believe him, and it filled my heart with joy.

He was delighted he had the chance to tell me thank you. I think it meant more to me than him, but from the looks of his smile, it may have been a tie. With a hug and a smile, I left his room, but he remained in my thoughts. Such a simple thing means a lot to each of us.

# *I WATCHED MY PATIENT GO TO HEAVEN*

**AFTER RECEIVING THE** report on this new patient, I walked into her room and she said she needed to go to the bathroom. She was extremely ill and exceptionally weak. I escorted her to the toilet after she refused a bedpan. After she washed her hands, I helped her back into bed. The tech had changed her sheets while we were in the bathroom, which was a pleasant surprise and refreshing.

I had a little trouble understanding her due to a language barrier. Then, in walked my favorite male tech, who was Hispanic. I told my tech that this patient was Spanish-speaking only and was there with terminal pancreatic cancer. Told him there were clean sheets, and I had just taken her to the bathroom. Her family was not here yet that morning as it was 6:30 a.m. So I brought him up to speed and turned around to leave the room.

Then, instantly, everything changed. She rejected everything and everyone around her. She kept pointing to the corner of the ceiling and outstretching her hands with her palms up. She would not let me or anyone touch her. She was rapidly talking and pleaded in Spanish. The patient kept on and on looking at the ceiling. The tech said, "She sees the angels, and she is telling them to take her to God." He went to her bedside, and she said, "Don't touch me. I am leaving." That was the last she acknowledged any of us in the room.

Instantly, I called her family and explained her quick change. I explained to them they should come in. She made a turn for the worse. Within minutes, the husband walked through the door. She had two sons, and I suggested the husband call them to come in. I was told in report that the family was very close. Within moments, the adult sons were there.

She continued looking at the ceiling and praying, remaining totally unaware of a presence of anyone except something in the corner of the ceiling. I felt badly that she did not acknowledge the boys or her husband. Not only did she not talk or look at them, but she vehemently refused their touch or closeness to the bed.

Her boys translated, saying Mom was holding an Angel's hand and saying, "thank you." "Please take me home" was her constant plea as she continued to focus on the ceiling. Then, she succumbed to a moment of peace and calm. The fight and pleas of desperation were gone. She calmly lay back in bed and closed her eyes. The son said, "The angel granted her wish."

I was pleased they all got to be with her and watch how peaceful everything was. I looked at her adoring family and said, "She is in Heaven now."

"Yes, we got to see her go, and this was her wish," said the husband. They were thankful to see how willing she was and how ready she was to leave her pain and suffering behind. Of course, they were sad and had their share of tears but also hung to the fact that yes, "Heaven and angels are real."

# WHEELCHAIR FOR SALE

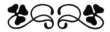

**AS A FAIRLY** new nurse, this day was a traumatic event for me. My patient had lost one leg last year to diabetes and vascular disease. Now, he was back to the hospital to have the other leg amputated.

I will never forget cleaning his remaining leg and prepping it for an amputation surgery. The thought of him returning to his room without a leg was almost unbearable for me. Not only are they removing his leg, but he lost his other one last year. How can you cut off a guy's leg? I was so glad not to have been the OR nurse. Knowing it was medically necessary and lifesaving was not enough to erase my seeing him leave the room. I was a new nurse and not prepared for the grim details of amputations.

I took a moment and went to the locker room to cry it out. And I thought I was strong. Well, I exposed my weakness that day. I tried to reason that it was a medical necessity, but that didn't help me. Literally my stomach churned all day. I wasn't sure I could handle this. As I held his leg, I realized it was cold. He also reacted to my touch while I was cleaning it with antiseptic and was as gentle as I could possibly be.

Watching him leave for the OR, I wasn't sure if I could emotionally adjust to this. It was a tremendously gruesome thought to know he would come back without a leg.

He returned to his room, and I realized it was the surgery that frightened me the most. His bandages were fresh and clean. There was no open gaping wound. It just looked like a support hose. My anxiety subsided, and I was able continue his care without hesitation. I realized what scared me was the thought of being in the OR and seeing the surgery.

Gone was the infected and painful part. I realized they just gave him more life to live and without pain. I grew up that day when I realized we are there for the good of the patient and not to promise more than we can deliver. We all made a difference that day, and I was at peace with that.

The following day was even a better day for me, and the patient was comfortable. He was preparing to return to his nursing home residence.

A social worker came in and told us they could not get him a wheelchair of his own and he would have to share with the others at his facility. Here was a double amputee with no personal wheelchair. I begged and pleaded but to no avail. They were not at fault. I was, for wanting what they tried but unable to get. This seemed totally inhumane. They were not trying to be mean or keep something from him. It was a matter of insurance and availability. My anxiety returned, but now I was focused on another issue, a wheelchair.

On my way home, I was still haunted by the situation. Truly mortified. Then, I saw there was a building on the corner with a sign: "Medical Equipment Supply Store." I pulled right in. My body and soul were determined. Told you I was stubborn, didn't I?

The store owner suffered through my pleas for a used wheelchair. He had some almost new-looking chairs, but I didn't even want to ask about them. This was a charity move on my part, and I guess I expected everyone to see it the way I did. I'm sure the store owner saw a determined nurse that was desperate to fix this.

The owner of the shop stated they did get an old wheelchair in yesterday. It was a little beat up and no fancy luxuries. It wasn't anything special, but he would sell it to me for $35. I had not given any consideration as to my financial ability to pay for this. It was obvious that was what he paid for it by the look on his face. I dug deep into every pocket and went to the car to check and see if I had anything. The best I came up with was a $10 bill and a $5 bill. After a pause, he smiled and said, "Would you like me to put it in your car?" Surely, he saw my excitement. Must have said thank you a million times.

The best $15 ever spent. Plus he probably has told that crazy nurse story to a lot of people. The chair looked as though it had been used hard. In people years, it looked like an 85-year-old without any cosmetic plastic surgery.

Quickly, I drove back to the hospital with my chair, feeling as though a monumental crisis had been averted. The receptionist confirmed the patient was still there and immediately took the chair to the patient. When she returned, she said, "He started crying when I told him, Someone dropped this off for you and wished to remain anonymous".

Nurses fix things that doctors can't control. Doctors fix things nurses can't, as well. That's why we are a team. I feel that I did my job that day. What a great feeling. The store owner did a great thing that day too. I sent him a thank-you note and told him about the patient's reaction.

We can all make a difference. Hospitals can't always fix every-thing, but they do go the distance for their patients. I've learned that hospitals are full of miracles and wishes. Sometimes they can come true in spite of hurdles. All we can do is try. And that, we did.

# *MAKING CHOICES*

**NURSING REQUIRES ONE** to be honest and strong. We always respond with the best interest of the patient in mind. We learn how, over time, to deliver news that is not always pleasant. Most of the time we are successful.

I loved being the nurse they chose to send to their anxious or demanding patients. Truth is that some patients needed honest, straight, and convincing conversations with someone with an ability to de-escalate issues. Being a patient or family member is very stressful emotionally, and so sometimes they react in irrational ways, which generally is due to lack of understanding or communication. Most of the time, they just want to be heard. I probably filled this qualification as I was older when I started nursing school. They did not see me as the "right out of school" nurse, and they probably thought I knew more than I did. Age or experience on the unit doesn't always mean qualified. What does matter is someone who can connect with patients and families who require a nurse that can solve difficult situations.

Mrs. Ann was in an accident that resulted in her being in a permanent coma. Fortunately, she was being well-cared for by her devoted daughter. Ann had remained in a coma for years, during which time her daughter was there every day to bathe her, curl her hair, turn her, supply silk pillow cases, polish her nails, apply makeup every day, bring special foam pillows to keep her heels up off the bed, and check on her hospital care as well. She had very high expectations, but I was happy to have her help, actually. We got along very well, and I was glad she requested me. I knew what she wanted, and she knew I would care for her mother. There were times when things did not go as planned, but we got along more like sisters, so we ended up laughing about the blips.

As a nurse, days don't always go smoothly. Every now and then, there are situations where emotions interfere with medical advice. Doctors will collect patient data and formulate a treatment plan according to the diagnostic needs.

One day, the daughter was told by the doctor that her mother needed a procedure due to her mom's labs being severely elevated. Her daughter declined, as she was afraid her mom would die if the necessary procedure was carried out.

Ms. Ann's daughter called me on the phone and proceeded to give me a long explanation of her fears and anger. It was obvious she was very worked up regarding the downturn situation that her mother was experiencing. Not once did I interrupt her passionate opinion. I gave her a chance to calm herself down. After asking her if she was done, I explained the risk her labs levels presented and the serious reaction it would cause to her body. Of course, she challenged me, and I answered all of her challenges with logical and documented medical reasons. I was calm through the entire conversation. Then followed up by letting her know, it was her decision to make and we would respect it.

Then, the conversation turned to me to explain and educate her on the what-if outcomes of each scenario.

I began by telling her how much I've enjoyed her mother and being given the privilege of taking care of her. It felt more like a family member. But I told her to think about how she would feel if she declined the procedure and her mother did not improve. A decline in her condition that may not be reversible. In fact she was already rapidly declining according to the doctors. The phone conversation went silent as I gave a pause in my talking. I wanted her to process her decision after being given all the facts. The doctor's had already told her all of this but I was only reminding her of that conversation. I encouraged her to weigh the possible consequences of each choice. I gave her one last chance to consider her choices and told her to think on it. But her immediate response was an emphatic *no*. Then, I conceded and told her I respected and understood the tough decision she had to make.

Bright and early the next day, I was working on another unit when she approached my desk. She started by saying, "I want to thank you, and I owe you an apology." I assured her none was needed and these are tough decisions when it is a family member. I added, I was only making sure she understood and of course the decision was her's to make". Later on the night, after I left my shift, her mother took a significant turn for the worse. The doctor had called the daughter to let her know she was critical, and the daughter promptly gave a go-ahead for treatment. She wanted to let me know her mom had the procedure that night and was doing fine. She told me they appreciated the honest and information I had given them and wished they would have said yes right then. She said, "You were right".

Families are faced with innumerable difficult decisions. Nurses just have to give them time to process and be strong for them in a calm way. It takes time to do this, but it's the right way for the patient and the family.

# A MOTHER'S LOVE

**A YOUNG MAN** had an accident, leaving him with a serious permanent head injury. He was a promising athlete and student. All of life to live was still ahead of him. Wonderful family. A mother with wishes for only the best things in life for her precious grown son. We never imagine anything but a good future for our children. I think our visions for them are even more grand than they can wish for. We plan their future from the day they are born. Never do we include obstacles that can derail the pathways of our hopes for them. As they grow, we increase the dreams, way beyond the ones they have. We think that they are 10 times more amazing than they think they are. You've heard the title, Mama Bear. Well, it is true. We never factor in anything for them except living the dreams they were born to live.

Her vision for him was one of joy and a successful future. He faithfully and diligently worked on his beloved sports all through high school and excelled as an athlete. In addition he was a great student. He also had a scholarship.

On one fateful day, all those dreams were instantly shattered. Mom was at his bedside and did not leave for days. She stood there frozen as a grief-stricken mother. She had been torn to pieces from the inside out and was forever crushed to her very core. Her soul nagged at her knowingly about the current situation, but she fought hard with more fiber and guts than I've ever witnessed. She refused to accept even the possibility of this being a lifelong sentence.

Mom was so proud of her son. You could see he was the most important thing in her life. She would have traded places gladly that very second if there was any way to accommodate that impossible exchange. She expressed this in every deep and labored breath she took plus every word she begged. Anxiety and disbelief caused her to engage in nonstop talking and reliving the good things he had done and things to come, which is a typical avoidance and a renunciation of situational facts. It took a lot of time letting her adjust to the picture now at hand and holding onto the memories of countless times of joy. She didn't want to let go of the dreams of his bright future. This is normal for any loving mother. The opposite would be cold and uncaring and unimaginable of any mom. The stages of grief are many and forever present. These stages don't carry an exact timetable.

The doctor walked and began to talk to the mother about the irreversible nature of her son's recent events. These words were not given with any harsh explanation. But I don't think the mother took one breath while the doctor was talking. Although, she heard these words before, Mom refused to associate them with the description of her son. To the mom this was fixable. But facts so move evidence of it not. Refusing to accept this assessment, the mother was thinking that, surely, the doctor was talking about the wrong patient, who was in the room next door. She was not ready to accept this cruel reality for her son. As a protective shield, we think if we don't accept it, it's not real. The doctor left, and the mother took another deep breath and told me to go fire that doctor and that he was never allowed to come back in this room.

Although the doctor was 100 percent right with all the information and did not present it in a harsh way, Mom wanted every bad and negative thing to be thrown out of the room. If we had incense to surround the room with, I think she would have tried that. Anything to ward off the pain or face reality. Maybe, her thoughts or hopes that a different doctor may have a better outcome.

I approached the doctor, then sitting at the nurses' station, putting in the daily note. Then, I said, "That was a really rough message to have to deliver." I proceeded to let the doctor know everything that was said was given in a gentle and as sugar-coated as possible. "But the patient wants to fire you as the doctor." Then a look of surprise came across his face. "I know this has nothing to do with you as a doctor," I tried to assure him. "She is just not ready to accept these facts of life. It's just you were the bad guy that had to deliver the news". I reminded him that he has a child about the same age. "Yes," was the response. "Just think how you would feel if someone, although truthful, gave you this grave news. You probably would medically understand and appreciate the facts being a doctor but would be upset also being a parent." His eyes reflected a better understanding when putting himself into this situation. "You just got her on a day she was not prepared for the reality, and that day may never come. Mom is not mentally well enough to accept this or anyone trying to tell her the real story. I told the doctor we just needed to give her time and inform the new doctor of the tender situation that exists for the mother. Perhaps I can ask the chaplain to come see her too."

My relationship with this doctor strengthened after this. He asked about this patient every time I saw him, not only concerned about the patient but the mother. Doctors do care, but we all get hit with bad timing from time to time, and this was just one of those. Actually, I don't think there would ever be a good time.

# *STRAIGHT TALK*

**EVERY DAY PRESENTS** its challenges. They are not always warm and fuzzy. There is no menu to choose from when we come to work. We are given a list of our patients, and their situations can change at a moment's notice. Strength and planning is required when one commits to doing the best for every patient. These challenges are generally explained before personally assessing a patient, giving us some time to think about the pros and cons that could arise upon one's first morning assessment. Plans are made as we consider possible red flags, thus being signs to watch that might reflect any negative conditions. And, we prepare as well as we can for these drastic fluid situations. There are always surprises every day.

My first patient of the day was a young man, 28 years old. I had this patient three months ago, and I remembered his case. Nothing had changed, except his condition had worsened. This cause for admission was completely self-inflicted after repeating the cause at will, a situation he was well-versed on and knew it would have a negative outcome if he persisted in repeating his past practices.

As I entered the room, the patient saw me and called me by name. "Hope that is a good memory, Mr. X," I responded. "Yeah, all's good. You're a nice nurse," he said. "Glad you think so because it's time for some straight mom talk. I'm going to be your best friend by telling you the truth straight up and without the coat of sugar." Then I began explaining to him, "You are a twenty-eight-year-old male, use cocaine, came in nine months ago due to overdose, stayed and recovered, and were sent home. Three months ago you came to the hospital in the exact same shape. Now, today, yep, you know, ditto." He was smiling which showed he still didn't grasp the gravity of this visit.

"Here is what you don't know. I don't judge you for your use of drugs. This is not meant to be a shaming session. This is a wake-up call that I think you need because I care about you. You're a good-looking guy and funny on top of that. You just aren't accepting that the car you are driving in does not have any brakes. You have worn out the brake pads. So the next time you drive down this road going 100 miles an hour, you probably won't be able to come back here to be saved. The sign you see will probably have the word 'END' on it." Like Dead End. He looked at me with a seriously frightened soul. He knew what I was saying. He wasn't angry; rather, he wanting to fix it and was ready to give me promises that only would sooth his mind but not prevent him from getting in that car (you understand my analogy, I hope). He was scared but not sure enough to stop.

I explained to him about his heart and how it was being deprived of what it needs: blood flow. The problem was called his heart's ejection fraction, the volume your heart can pump out each time it beats. The normal EF (ejection faction) is about 65 percent. This is with a healthy heart and gets lower when your heart fails to be strong enough to beat as needed. The pump fails. The heart's main function as a muscle is to pump blood throughout the body. When it weakens, we call this heart failure. The words are descriptive enough. Below are his percentages of blood his heart pumped was calculated on each of his visits. This raw fact, he understood.

First visit: 60%
Second visit: 40%
Now: 30%

"This heart failure is being contributed to your cocaine drug choice that you are making. I'm not saying you should substitute another drug, but the choice you made was the worst one you could have for your heart. We can only turn you back around so many times, and I think this is your last time to make a personal decision: What is more important, your life or your addiction? I don't think if you don't change, I'll be seeing you again. The numbers tell the story and not something I made up. If your heart doesn't pump, you don't live, and you're running on as close to empty as possible.

"There are heart transplants; however, as a drug abuser, you would most probably not be a candidate. I can't say for sure, but the possibilities would be slim, as there is a long waiting list, I know."

He was totally quiet and did not utter a word during my explanation. I let him process what I had told him. Then, he looked at me with wide eyes like those of a small child who had just seen a scary movie. I took his hand and said, "You can turn this around. I know you can. It will be the toughest thing you ever do, but if you want to, you can." He agreed to have a counselor see him. The counselor responded quickly to my page and arrived shortly afterward.

There was little conversation with him the rest of the day as he was back and forth in tests, counseling, and procedures. We did not have much time in-between other activities.

Before my shift ended, I returned to his room one last time. "Mr. X, it's your turn to tell me how you are doing. My hopes are that today has been a leap in the right direction for you. Do you want to share your thoughts with me?" He started crying and immediately my apology was forthcoming. "I'm sorry to have been so straight with you. It does you no good for me to be dishonest." He proceeded to tell me about his visit with the counselor and thanked me for being there for him. He said, "You are still a nice nurse and I'm going to try. They have already set up counseling for me," he softly said. I gave him a hug and said, "Hey, it's gonna be tough, but I think you are worth saving."

I gave one last glance back to make sure he had a smile, and he did. "The next time I see you in here is when you bring me your smile and a plate of frosted cookies. None with a bite out of them, OK?"

I knew the odds were probably against him at this point. The fact that I never saw him again was somewhat sad, but my hopes drifted to a positive life change for him. This is a tough and nearly impossible addiction to beat.

# *"I KNOW"*

**THE ROOM SMELLED** like fresh vanilla. The mood was tranquil but not somber. My patient was lying in his bed asleep, and four family members were sitting in chairs by his bed. Their conversations felt happy, as evidenced by the smiles on their faces and their normal tone of voices. Once they noticed me entering the room, they stood up to greet me with hugs and appreciation. There wasn't a shred of gloom or doom. There wasn't that normal intense feeling or sense via verbal or visual acknowledgment of the serious condition of their father/grandfather. Contentment surrounded the room from corner to corner. Instantly, I became part of the cordial and welcoming mood as they had given me a sense of peace. Their comfort was contagious.

This is how consequential each of us can be to one another. It was not as though they scripted this aura. However, it became apparent to me that this was a natural state of living for this lovely family. Even their disagreements must have been dignified while maintaining the strength and principles to which they subscribed without falter.

As I approached the bedside quietly and without even a stir in the air, the patient opened his eyes and gave me a smile. I likened his smile to that of my grandfather, a Baptist minister. This was instantly personal for me, as I saw the gracious soul of a great man lying before me. Before I could formulate any words, he said, "I know." It wasn't until later that I understood what he meant.

This room became my retreat whenever I had a moment in the day. It was my time in which I was able to recharge myself and reflect on a way to help my other patients, who are not all this easy to be with. I understood they needed me more, but I needed the family and their embrace. We learn to gain strength and deliver strength throughout the day. They were my charging station, so to speak.

While caring for the patient, it was common knowledge that he was terminal. The patient and the family were very open and accepting of the limited time that awaited him here on earth. He always held my hand when I came in and then kissed the top of it when I let go to leave. He had a wink after that kiss, and I felt as though my father was giving me that wink. It was as if he knew me.

My last room to say goodnight to was of course my retreat room. The family was just getting ready to leave and were about to offer prayers. "Please come join us," they offered. Without hesitation, I stepped beside the family members and prayed my own silent prayer of thanks for this beautiful family. I felt like that six-year-old little girl I once was, who just wanted to be loved and not scolded.

My drive home was a peaceful moment. I felt shielded by their love. They gave me the energy to pass this love onto others. I wish I could convey to you how amazing this family was and is. There are no words that can describe unconditional love the way their actions did.

In an attempt to explain: You know that one person you can always count on. That one who at Christmas doesn't get you the biggest or most expensive present or the one on your list of made-up wants. He would be the one that got you a present that you would treasure forever, the present you didn't even know you wanted or needed, but it meant more than buying everything in any catalog I ever saw. What an amazing gift. He gave a gift of self and acceptance. We can give gifts like this every day. I say, make a habit of it.

On day two, I was looking forward to visiting their family. I arrived to work a half hour early. I walked into his room, and the family was surrounding his bed and holding hands. I froze. Tears welled up in my eyes. I knew what this must mean. "NO," I said to my heart, trying to ward off the possibility of him dying in the night. Even though he had not been begging for more time, I was. I stood at the door trying to gain enough courage to be strong and not selfish or needy.

Then, the daughter turned around and smiled. "Come on in and join us," she said. She opened up the circle, giving me a spot right next to his face. I braced myself and tried to muster enough self-control to not cry like a baby. As I connected my hands with the group, he turned his head and looked at me. That smile followed by that special wink made me almost collapse to the floor in wonder. My emotions were having difficulty in keeping up with the instant flip-flops they were enduring. A little tear trickled down my cheek, which I thought would be less noticeable than wiping it away, was not missed by my patient as it was by all the others who had their eyes closed. He was watching me as I was watching him. When the prayer was over, I stayed by his bedside, and he softly whispered, "I know." I shook my head in agreement as I knew he felt my thoughts even before I could have them. He spoke other words but these were of special meaning to both of us.

I don't know how I could have endured my day had he been gone. So my energy was put to work toward all my other patients in a way that had ever had more meaning. This is what I am destined to do, and what a wonderful gift I have been given. My job is to make lives better in any way that I can. I too can try to give back and trust that I can be at least a fraction of what I've learned.

Before I left for the evening, I stopped to say good night and that I would be back tomorrow. They invited me in for their family night prayer. Finally, I too was not afraid or sad anymore. He had lived a long life. His family was the picture of perfection. His love and devotion was going to live on, and hopefully, I can learn by his example and serve others.

Day three was the day for discharge. The family chose a wonderful nursing facility for him. What makes it perfect is the fact that I know they will still be there for him, and he will get the care he deserves.

Mid-morning, the daughter came out to the nurses' station and gave me a book, *Jesus Calling*. In the front, they wrote a very special thank-you note to me with wishes for my life ahead.

The time came for discharge. Interestingly, I was not sad. I was filled with a grateful heart. They pulled his wheelchair around the nurses' station and were headed to the elevator but stopped to say goodbye. I stood in front of him and bent down to cradle his face in my hands and kissed his forehead and told him, "I loved every minute with you and your family. I'll see you again someday, so save me a seat, OK?" He responded with, "I will," a wink, and as he looked into my eyes, he said, "I know." And that, he did.

I returned to the nurses station to write my final patient notes, when a co-worker asked me, "Are they family?" I responded with a smile and said, "Yes". But, my heart said they are even more.

# I GAVE MYSELF PERMISSION TO BREAK THE RULES

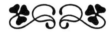

**ICU HAS STRINGENT** rules for a reason, and these rules are important to be followed in order to give the critically ill patients all the attention and constant care they need without interruptions. As a nurse, it is a commitment toward focus on only one thing, the patient. I respected and followed these rules as I pledged to do.

However, It is a hard rule to follow when the nurse's heart takes over. Yes, I broke a rule.

In the first room inside the door to the ICU lay a very young mother who was hooked up to every tube, IV drip, and oxygen mask in an effort to save her life. My desk was next to the waiting room door that had a small window. This gave me an unobstructed view where I could see the grandmother and daughter patiently waiting. Grandma had brought every distraction she could think of to occupy this adorable eight-year-old as Grandma awaited her abbreviated allowed visits. When it was time for the next visit, I opened the door and allowed my patient's mother to enter. It about broke my heart but the 8 yo daughter patiently remained seated due to ICU age restrictions. My patient was on isolation but this didn't prevent her mom from blowing kisses and giving smiles that were exchanged through a large window view into her daughter's room . All the while this sweet little gal sat in the waiting room playing with the toys her grandmother had so thoughtfully packed. During these moments, I took her cookies and sometimes just stepped out to talk to her. She always was polite and said thank you each and every time.

Shortly after visiting hours ended for the day, my heart could not stand it anymore. Seeing that angel sit there all day was too much. I went to the waiting room and asked the little princess if she would like to see her mom. A smile occupied that sweet face and she said yes, as she looked at grandma for permission.

I explained she would see her through a window, but she was not limited to the number of kisses she could blow to her or and the smiles she could exhibit. I said, "We need to put a smile on your mom's face. No tears, you need to be strong for your mommy."

I slid a chair up to the window so she could see her mom. They both waved and blew kisses. Then, without coaching, our little one made funny faces making us all realize what an unforgettable and very special moment we were experiencing. Then, it was time to say goodnight, so I picked her up and carried her high enough so she could see and wave to her mom until we walked out of the doors of the ICU. She wasn't sad. She was all childish giggles and made fun of mom's mask and tubes. I'm sure she still remembers that day—I do.

The next day, I was informed my patient had died early this morning. Although I was sad, I was glad to have allowed a little girl to see her mom one last time. As a nurse, sometimes our hearts lead us toward our loving instincts. It wasn't about following the general rules, it was about doing the loving thing at a time when time was limited. Those monkey faces were proof enough for me that this was one of those times. I think the hospital would have agreed this was the right thing to do. After all, God told me to do it.

# *GIFTS OF CARING ARE PRICELESS*

**THE BEST AND** most meaningful gifts are those that don't require money. Remember as a child picking a dandelion flower and giving it to your mom? The joy was in seeing her face light up as if this was the most precious things she ever got. And, truth be known, it was precious to her. You thought enough of her to make her happy and you wanted to give her something that would do just that. I'm a mom and I can assure you, this is a special moment.

Friendship is a gift showing someone cares about and will be there for you. Smiling is a gift that helps remind others there is good in life and is usually reciprocated with a smile confirming your gift was received and welcomed. Hugs, provide a feeling of closeness and belonging. A Wink, is flirtatious or sign of approval. Thank You, is a gift of appreciation. Holding A Door for someone is a gift of respect and kindness. Sending a Card or Letter is a gift of thoughtfulness and shows you took time to do something meaningful for someone else. None of these cost anything. It only takes a moment of caring enough to be thankful.

I could fill numerous pages with all the ideas and ways we can give the gift of love and kindness to others. A purchased gift is given in love and enjoyed while generally reserved for a special occasion. Note to husbands: don't forget those special occasions.

I'm just pointing out there are more ways to show others they matter and that is through a life of caring. Gifts from the heart.

Every day, I make a sincere effort to approach life with a smile and offer help wherever I am able. Gifts should never be given with expectations of an even exchange. The joy of giving is our immediate reward. And, what a wonderful feeling that is.

My work at the hospital was fulfilling, difficult, exhausting, and I wouldn't have traded it for the world. I was exposed to people in need of care on a daily basis and my gift was caring for each one of them.

One of my favorite days was when the University professors would bring their senior students in to experience floor time at a hospital. The nurses were given the option of having a student shadow or not. I never refused. As a matter of fact I was known to have at least one and most often 2 students. Absolutely loved seeing their inquisitive eyes filled with joy along with a tense feeling of being overwhelmed.

I remembered MY tough preceptor and how I felt when she would harshly point out my every flaw and shake her head. It was so intimidating because I really wanted to be good at what I did. She turned me loose with no real direction, then only to criticize me in front of my patients. I vowed to never treat a student nurse that way. I kept my promise. I wanted them to be as good as they can be.

Each student had a hands-on experience and learned the routines of being a good nurse. First rule, know the patient before you enter their room. Diagnosis, meds, vitals, procedures done or pending. I firmly stressed they need to be confident when they enter the room. Never answer any of their patient's questions with, "I don't know". Say, "Let me check the chart and make sure, or Dr. XXX will be rounding and I will definitely let Dr. XXX know you have a question or concern about that. I can then help you outside the room with the answer if I can and you can follow up with the patient. Prompt follow up with the patient is also one of the many Golden Rules. They need to have complete faith in their nurse and knowing they communicate with the doctors is a strong point in the plus column. It's a team effort.

The student's gift to me was at the end of their day when they said thank you and gave me a hug of appreciation and gratitude for helping show them the real life side of nursing. Made the effort well worth it.

Numerous years latter I moved to a different department in the hospital. A pleasant lady came up to me and called me Pam. Her face was familiar but I just couldn't place how we knew each other. Well, she didn't forget. I had been the nurse she shadowed as a student nurse. She told me how nervous she was and how she lacked confidence. Plus it was her brief time with me that gave her the courage to believe in her own abilities and have the confidence that let her be a good nurse.

These are the thank you notes that mean more than a gold watch or plaque for the wall. For her to remember me after all those years and be kind enough to tell me how special it was for her was precious to me.

As I watched her with others, I witnessed a kind and selfless person. A genuine giver. She had just given me a compliment that filled me with pride and purpose. This is a great example where one act of kindness can encourage and help another have the confidence to achieve their hopes and dreams. We can have a positive impact on someone just by showing a little kindness. As you can see, it only takes one person to give you hope and caring to change/improve your life.

Now, it was my turn to show her how special she is. Lunch seemed the perfect way to get to know each other outside of work.

A couple weeks latter we met at a Bonefish Grill for a bite to eat and enjoy some non business time together. When she walked in she was wearing her prettiest jewelry, her smile. I am old enough to be her mother but I thought maybe that is why we need to share some time together. We were comfortable in telling our stories since our past days. Now she was all grown up and had 5 children. The floodgates of our lives opened as we told the good and the difficult times during our journeys. The minutes turned into hours without a dull or uncomfortable second.

We have been good friends since that day. She is a treasured gift to me and I love hearing her stories of her adventures. And, it all began because of one small effort, a thank you.

Know when you give the gift of love and kindness, you may never be told how much it meant to that person. However, know this, you planted a seed of love and kindness. We can only trust that seed will grow and become another gift that will be passed along. If you only plant one seed of kindness a day, that's 365 seeds a year. Impressive right?

# IT TAKES A TEAM

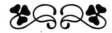

**HEALTHCARE IS A** Team Sport. As I have mentioned, I grew up with an "I Can Do It Myself" attitude. Then I grew up and realized everything in life is a team sport. Experience helped me realized how much of life is a collaborative effort if we want to be successful. A marriage, football, putting a man on the moon, parenting, and basically anything we become successful in has been possible because of a team effort with contributions from others. My revised slogan: I Can Do This with the help of others.

It takes a team. Doctors and nurses each serve an important function. Our desired collaborative outcome is the same but our roles differ. Using a football analogy, the quarterback is a highly important player on the team but is not solely responsible in taking the football all the way to the goalpost.

I've talked a lot about the interactions a nurse has with a patient. However, the doctor is the quarterback that hands that patient to the nurse to help get them to the goalpost.

Sometimes our roles give the appearance that one team member cares more than another. Just when you think that, you are proven wrong. Everyone of us cares a great deal. Our duties dictate our main focus of responsibilities.

There is a doctor that comes to mind when I think of focus. I shall refer to him as Dr. Focus. His skills are exceptional. He always took on the most difficult cases. Amazing is the word that flashes through my head when I think of all the patients that are alive today because of his commitment to his professional skills.

He was not the person who would stand and chat up a conversation next to the water cooler. He was completely immersed in the care of the patient. He was always what I would call, laser focused. I was constantly intrigued by his commitment and vast knowledge. Yes, he had lots of Ego and I believed he earned every ounce of it and it was not just self ordained because of a degree.

The key is, as a nurse, we have a job to do. Our job is to apply our own laser focus on the patient to ensure an optimal outcome when the patient is assigned to us. We also jump in to help other nurses when needed.

Jason, a new patient was a young man with a lovely wife and a 5 y.o. child . He won the lottery in my mind to have Dr. Focus as his doctor. I was given this patient to care for the moment he left the recovery room. All was going well.

When I arrived the next day, this patient was gone and I assumed he had been downgraded to a lower level of care.

Within a couple hours into my shift at work, in walks the surgeon and onto the floor. He looked like he'd slept in his clothes and his hair looked similar to that of a child who just came in off the playground. I greeted him with a good morning and he looked at me with eyes burdened from exhaustion and pain.

"Pam, can I see you for a moment"?

"Sure", I said as I followed him into a vacant patient's room. One look at him and I was sure he was about to deliver the bad news of our patient not living through his surgery.

I just stood there numb as I was looking at him. A man who always dressed meticulously, now stood before me, looking as though he just awakened from a park bench after spending the night on it.

"I've been up all night. We took Jason downtown last night. He was rejecting the graft I put in." Dr. Focus felt the pain of his own words and allowed his vulnerable side to surface. A few tears began to role down his cheeks as he turned away from me. "We took him back to surgery and were able to fix the bleeding that had sprung forth. I stayed by his bedside through the night watching him to make sure everything would be ok. He made it but I was really upset", he confessed. This was real life evidence of how every bit of this man's sole is 100% wrapped up in his patients.

Here was a doctor who was always calm, controlled, and determined. He was exposing his typically concealed, fragile, emotional side to a select audience of just Me. I got him a cool washcloth and told him how special he is. Plus I told him how proud we all were of him every day. This was no exception. He was who he always is, there for the patient and bringing his excellent talents to each and every one of them.

After a small up turned hint of a smile, he took a full deep breath and left to do what he does best. Save Lives. We never mentioned that day again, but I never saw him but when I didn't think, there goes our hero.

# KUDOS, PATIENT CARE TECHS

**SENDING OUT A** special thanks to the patient care techs I personally worked with and all those who were there for all the patients and nurses.

A nursing team is a group of trained professionals that work toward a common goal. Our team assignment is to take care of patients. We perform together like a family away from home. Our mission is a shared responsibility to which we count heavily on one another. Some days we acquire additional duties, which generates more stress. We depend on our team to lend extra support where needed. We all dig deep to find the energy to perform an addition to an already exhausting group effort. Situations in the hospital can change quickly making a small task an all consuming one. We stand ready to meet those needs. Without our team, we would not be able to give our patients or each other the support that is needed.

One of the team's biggest support system is that of the job of our Techs. Techs set up meal trays, wash patients, change gowns, change sheets, clean up after bouts with nausea, take care of the bedpan, chart vitals, and chart I&Os, walk patients, most of them with pumps and poles attached to them, turn patients in bed, get ice, refill water pitchers, comb hair, adjust pillows, and report to nurses any changes in patient noted. Please forgive me if I've failed to mention the other 1,000 things you do. But you get the picture. However, you'd have to be there to understand the hectic pace in the day to day life of a Tech and the Nurses.

Nurses really appreciate you, even though we sadly seldom take the time to thank you enough. Unfortunately and unintentionally, we sometimes fail to verbalize praise for what our techs manage to achieve each day. Our failure is in not seeing what is done but only seeing what is not done. So we lean on them with a negative tone and not enough on the positive. Our daily tasks demand a lot from us as well. However, without you, we couldn't do it.

I personally, could not have done my job without each one of you. I send a heartfelt thank-you to everyone I've ever worked with and every tech who works in any hospital: Job well done!

# PSYCHOLOGY CLASS

**PSYCHOLOGY CLASS WAS** not only about reading our assignments and taking a test on the subject matter discussed in the chapters. Our tenured professor was passionate about her profession. Her belief was more about observing related behaviors. Cues are hints and serve as missing puzzle pieces shown by the patient's choice of words, body movements, eye positions, and key words that changed behavior. Communication is an observation sport. It was a class filled with more questions than answers: listening, watching, using provocative words, and introspection.

We were provided real-case studies of several types of mental illnesses. Not only were we able to read about the case, but we were given the opportunity to see these patients during a group session. Books can provide definitions, but the real-life cases provide a relatable visual, helping us experience a better understanding. Visits to various mental health facilities provided us with real-life examples of patients who suffer from various mental illnesses and drug addiction.

A trip to our first facility was to a drug rehab for adults. While sitting in on group counseling sessions, we were encouraged to witness the responses among the patients as well as verbal redirection responses when asked questions from the therapist. All of these real-life scenarios afforded us a personalized picture into the many diagnosis types researched in our classes. We were tasked with identifying a diagnosis of each of the patients. We did not interact but only observed. My curiosity focused on the therapist's response to the patient's body language, not only their verbal language. She maneuvered the mine fields and buried treasures like the pro she was.

With only two more weeks of class, we were given a term paper assignment. "This is your last test," she said, with a small pause. I suspected she expected a loud clamor of excitement. Strangely, the room was silent. She stated, "Your assignment is to write a term paper on what you learned in class and how the experience will impact your nursing career." There were some grumbles, but I was excited as I had already formed an opinion on psych nursing. The part I was missing was the part where she said how it will impact *my* nursing career. Psychology has a way of making us think about the not so obvious. I had no idea on how this could help until later on in my nursing career, when I realized I used my learning every day. It helped me to understand my patients better.

At first, the class had no interest to me. And honestly, I think I have realized in writing this book that I used her theories and cues and silence to learn more about a patient than I would have without them. She made a difference in my understanding, and I learned a little patience as well.

This paper came before I matured as a nurse. I now look back on her response to it and say, "She had my attention by accepting me for who I was and yet, leaving an impression to be a better me at who I wanted to be not only in healthcare but in life."

# PSYCHOLOGY TERM PAPER

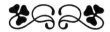

**THIS WAS THE** easiest paper I ever wrote. Can you believe I wrote a paper trashing my professor's nursing field choice and passion—one she obviously excelled in and had a total connection with? Her dedication was so real and natural as if these patients were her kids.

Never once did I think about appeasing her. I only thought of myself and how this area of nursing was a hard *no* for me. I wrote feverishly and fluidly about the anxiety and depression I witnessed each day during the facility visits. Now, I took on those feelings and found it difficult to deflect them. I wrote how sad it made me feel and what my unspoken response was toward working with this, day-in and day-out. The anxiety of it all was disturbing to me. On and on, I went relentlessly. From the notes I took during these sessions, I detailed specific moments that were unlike the world I was accustomed to. How disturbing it was that people lived in these weighty mental capsules of turmoil.

Without hesitation, I turned in the paper a day early. In fact, the next day. I was proud of what I wrote, but after I turned it in, I started questioning what her response would be. Is this an insult to her? Would she think I didn't understand the course material? Was she ready to hear negative personal thoughts from my gut?

My psychology professor was an uplifting person. I think she knew me better than I knew myself. No, I know she did. Without a doubt, she would love to see what I am writing now after applying her class lessons in psychology. All along she was bringing me out by allowing me to express myself. She gave my feelings permission to be visited and pondered. All this without ridicule or harsh judgement. More than I did when judging her professional choice. Or so I thought. In hindsight, I feel she would think this was not criticism but more about understanding myself and allowing me to express what I like and don't like.

Now, what I realize is that every student was in counseling while attending her class. Can you imagine being her child? Just kidding but the thought has crossed my mind. She probably was an amazing mother. In her class, the students did most of the talking that was spontaneously provoked by her questions. This was so subtle I'm not sure everyone saw it, but we had exposed ourselves through our conversations. She would gently give meaning to the unresolved hurts and anger several were experiencing. We began to identify with her examples and truly saw the rawness of these wounds from our lives. She provided a punctuation to learning through her delicately and totally thoughtfully presented class discussions. Soon, she knew us better than we knew ourselves. Then she gave us the gift of understanding ourselves. It was like a personal introduction into knowing who we are and why we feel the way we do. We were given permission to feel this way, and it also provided avenues we could take to become what we wanted to be and feel, all along abandoning our guilt and retiring our anger by parking some of it on the other side of the street.

We all learned more than most of us realized was possible. Thus, we became a better form of ourselves. It was not until I began writing this book that I understood how much her teaching and insight helped me be the nurse that I became. I soon embraced the unique and various passions, likes, dislikes, talents, and challenges life brings to each of us. The calico quilt of life is complex and no two are alike. If we listen, we can better understand where the pain comes from in people. When they have an outlet granted to release their pain, we know better how to be there for them. The sad hard truth, however, is when we realize we cannot fix everything or everyone, but we can show some comfort through compassion along the way.

Then I used her teaching insights every day in some way to help my patients and into my extended journey. All of this is through applying pieces and parts of what I learned and is a result of her compassion and nonjudgmental approach to teaching. It wasn't until years later, as I reflected on her class, that I realized that wounds are not all visible. We can put on Band-Aids, do surgery, give medication, but this does not heal the invisible wounds held deep within their hearts and minds. Some wounds happened yesterday and some, many years ago.

A kind gesture mixed with some compassion prove to be an important practice. Don't get me wrong, I was a strong nurse and have had some tough talks with my patients, but the combination created a bond of respect. Permission to express feelings affects healing considerably more than we realize. You don't have to be a nurse to fill or use this script for compassion. It's not required by the FDA.

To my surprise, I got an A+ on my term paper, followed by this note: "Beautifully Written." I felt recognized for being me and it was OK.

After class, I confessed to her my angst after writing my true, raw reaction slamming the profession she dearly loves. I thought maybe she'd be insulted.

She smiled and responded with: "Being able to understand and know yourself and others is what this course was about. You absolutely captured the vision of this class."

She had given me permission to express my true feelings without punishment, in turn, learning the joy of giving others the same permission to be themselves. It doesn't get any better than this.

# ALWAYS LEAVE SOMETHING GOOD OF YOURSELF BEHIND

**ALTHOUGH MY NURSING** career has run its course, every day is a new opportunity to grow into a new and improved version of myself. A résumé is not something we are born with nor is it completed at any set time in life. My glass is still only half full, and I intend to keep on and have the joy of adding more to it every day, then seeing it overflow. If it does, I'm going to get a bigger glass.

Every day I am blessed with the opportunity to embrace a new journey. I don't want to be someone else—I know that job has been taken. Where is the adventure and pride in making copies? Grow to acquire those new strengths, and become a blended version of yourself. My advice is to never make excuses nor accept them. Never look strictly for success. If you are upgrading or embellishing your journey, start looking for what makes you happy within yourself. You can admire someone, but you can't be them; however, you can be a better version of yourself and own something special that you can be proud of. Seeking happiness does not mean that is all that will happen along your journey. An oops will appear along your way. I truly hope you find it in yourself to shake your head and laugh at yourself. This is called learning and does not mean this roadblock is a dead end. Keep some lead in your pencil, and make sure it has a good eraser. You will find this beneficial. Sounds easy, right? Well, writing it is easier than living it, but I've lived to have many new journeys, and believe me, it's been worth the struggles and rewrites of my life.

Live fearlessly. If you open door #1, and it's not the grand prize, open door #2, then door #3. Eventually, you will find what you are looking for. There are many doors of opportunities out there. Never give up. See ,think, dream, plan, then go for it with a childlike innocence, trust, and determination.

Make a note to yourself: first, if you fall, remember to get back up.

My motto, one of many that I make up to fit the situation: "Treat yourself to a cookie occasionally, vegetables wilt." A cookie will be there waiting for you. Or, you can make more. They have a way of loving you back. Remember, if you eat it alone, you don't have to feel guilty.

Never build your journey on jealousy. Jealousy provokes resentments and bad behavior from all parties involved. Instead, build it out of respect and acknowledge verbally your admiration of said qualities. Be selective and learn to incorporate that which you find positive and useful for your growth while serving as a good example to others. Beware, there are takers in relationships. Try to avoid being one who solely takes. Blend your life with giving. There is more than a one-size journey. Looks good on some but does not fit everyone. Find what you value in your life, and tailor it to fit you. Then wear it with pride. Even those who graduated at the top of their class, trust me, they still have a lot of stuff to learn. When we start thinking we know it all, we stop learning and become obsolete. That sounds a little too lonely for me.

Surround yourself with those you admire, those smarter, more experienced, and be excited for what they know. They are the ones you can learn the greatest amount from. Most will be so flattered for their recognition of their talents, they will gladly be your coach. Fortunately, I learned at a very early age to latch onto the kites of those with a wealth of knowledge. Remember, they had teachers too. Knowledge is not a present someone can bestow upon us at birth. This practical understanding took them years to learn, so listen and soar in the vacuum of their sails. Position yourself beside the best of the best. Watch, listen, look, and follow your thirst for learning. Downside, they may be a little too self-loving, but I didn't say you had to share an apartment—I said: learn. Warning: don't strive to be them, but strive to be a better you.

Some of the best advice I ever got is that every job you have will become a portrait of yourself. Autograph it with an honest effort and excellence. Quality is an act of doing the right thing even when there are no spectators. You never know when there might be someone peeking around the corner.

The pride of accomplishment you possess will be felt every day. Give it your unyielding desire, willingness to learn, be part of the team, plus sprinkle on some glitter of laughter to make your personal light shine. Remember this golden rule, store-bought maps are only suggested routes. You can glance at them to make sure you are headed in the right direction, but remember this is your life. Follow your heart's detour, and draw your personal side road maps to fulfill dreams along the way. Maps usually suggest the easiest routes, the fastest from point A to B. But remember, there are a lot of sites to see off the major highway. Embrace a few detours, and enjoy the beauty of life. Take off your sunglasses and let in the beauty of the mountains and rivers. Those who follow the turnpikes only see concrete and will miss the sunflowers in bloom, the cows with a young calf, the waterfalls, the church spire and echoing of its bell, the kids playing hop scotch, the joyful excitement of puppies meeting other puppies while being walked, the sound of crickets in the thick of the willow trees and moss blowing in the wind, two people hugging under the dim night light, a mother pushing a stroller, and so much more. We were given eyes to see beauty, so don't miss it. Like the cookies I highly suggested, these, too, are sweet things in life. Taste them whenever possible. They also bring us back to our humble selves and slow our breathing enough to relax and smell the precious memories of childhood.

Continue to strive and be a person who delivers more positivity than negative chaos. Set your goals. If your chosen road leads you away from your desires, fill up with gas and reroute. Goals can be adjusted, so make sure they are preferably in a positive direction.

Life is your gift, so unwrap it with love, and you will be astounded with the gifts you may find inside. Life is not about warming yourself by the fire—it is about building that fire. Think of yourself as the match that ignites your dreams, then bask in the warmth and glow.

# POINT YOUR TOES FORWARD

**THROUGH LIFE I'VE** carried three-by-five cards with inspirational sayings on them. I refer to them during moments when I can only see the darkness and the clouds. I read them, but do I follow them to the letter? No. Plus I don't expect you to follow my suggestions to the tee either. These are my road maps and the cheat sheets to my life. They too can survive detours.

I hope and pray that you find/found your happy places in life, having fulfilled the most incredible journey you can even imagine and beyond, and with much more to come. Don't forget to look back and relive life so you can truly celebrate the people, the towns, the events, and those whom have served as an inspiration. I wish you every possible accomplishment you strive for in your life along your chosen journeys.

Thank you for letting me share my stories with you. My wish for you is that you have received inspiration for your road map that will fulfill every dream of yours in the days ahead. We just need the courage sometimes to turn our backs on disappointments and *point your toes forward*.

Printed in the USA
CPSIA information can be obtained
at www.ICGtesting.com
CBHW072050110124
3289CB00002B/10

9 781662 889400